IBS Relief

IBS Relief

A Complete Approach to Managing
Irritable Bowel Syndrome

UPDATED AND EXPANDED EDITION

DAWN BURSTALL, R.D., M.H.S.A.
T. MICHAEL VALLIS, PH.D.
GEOFFREY K. TURNBULL, M.D.

WILEY

John Wiley & Sons, Inc.

Published by John Wiley & Sons, Inc., Hoboken, New Jersey
Published simultaneously in Canada

The questionnaire on page 11 was adapted with permission from "Appendix B: Rome II Modular Questionnaire: in *Rome II: The Functional Gastrointestinal Disorders* by D.A. Drossman, et al. © 2000 Degnon Associates (www.romecriteria.org). All rights reserved

Illustrations in chapter 3 by Geoffrey K. Turnbull

The information contained in this book is not intended to serve as a replacement for professional medical advice. Any use of the information in this book is at the reader's discretion. The author and the publisher specifically disclaim any and all liability arising directly or indirectly from the use or application of any information contained in this book. A health care professional should be consulted regarding your specific situation.

For general information about our other products and services, please contact our Customer Care Department within the United States at (800) 762-2974, outside the United States at (317) 572-3993 or fax (317) 572-4002.

Wiley also publishes its books in a variety of electronic formats. Some content that appears in print may not be available in electronic books. For more information about Wiley products, visit our web site at www.wiley.com.

Library of Congress Cataloging-in-Publication Data:

Burstall, Dawn.
  [I.B.S. relief]
  IBS relief : a complete approach to managing irritable bowel syndrome / Dawn Burstall,
  T. Michael Vallis, and Geoffrey K. Turnbull.—2nd ed.
     p. cm.
  Includes index.
  ISBN-13 0-978-0471-77547-8 (pbk.)

  1. Colon (Anatomy)—Diseases. 2. Irritable colon—Alternative treatment.
I. Vallis, T. Michael. II. Turnbull, Geoffrey K.   III. Title.
RC862.I77B87 2006
616.3'42—dc22

2005029363

10 9 8 7 6 5 4

To Dr. Ronald T. Tanton, a gastroenterologist of superior clinical acumen whose mentoring encouraged us to develop our team approach.

Contents

Acknowledgments

We wish to thank the many people under our care who have taught us about treating irritable bowel, and in so doing, have helped us share this knowledge with you. As well, we would be remiss if we did not thank our colleagues. They facilitated our collaboration, which led to the development of this treatment plan by encouraging an approach to patient care that includes doctors, dietitians, and psychologists working together.

On a more personal note, Dawn thanks Bob Kelly, who encouraged and supported her throughout this project. Michael thanks his daughter, Emily, for her support and encouragement. Geoff thanks his wife, Patty, for her encouragement throughout this project. Thanks also to Ben for his support and encouragement. Special mention goes to Katie, who worked tirelessly with her dad to bring this book to fruition.

Introduction

For two weeks now, you've had daily episodes of diarrhea, abdominal pain so severe you can't think straight, and stomach bloating. You are afraid to eat and can hardly venture out of sight of a bathroom (twice in the past three days you've barely made it). You know something is seriously wrong, but your doctor—who just returned your second call of the week—says the test results confirm her impression: there is nothing wrong with you. How can this be? You know what you feel. You're terrified it might be serious (cancer), but you can't talk to your friends about your bowels.

If this sounds familiar, this book is for you.

We are a team of health professionals (a clinical nutritionist, a health psychologist, and a gastroenterologist) who treat individuals with irritable bowel at a gastroenterology clinic in a large urban teaching hospital. We have developed a treatment plan based on the current scientific knowledge about irritable bowel, nutrition, stress, and coping. The purpose of this book is to provide a how-to manual so that you can do this treatment on your own. Like most things in life, there is an upside and a downside to this.

The upside is: this is a how-to manual that will help you manage irritable bowel. The methods that you will learn in this book are based on scientific studies showing that the methods are effective in improving irritable bowel symptoms. If you follow this workbook closely, there is good reason to expect that your symptoms will improve.

The downside is: this is a how-to manual that will help you manage irritable bowel. The very thing that makes this workbook helpful is also the thing that makes this book a challenge: it is a how-to manual that requires you to do the work. This is not the kind of book that you can just read and put aside. If you want this book to help you, you need to be prepared to do some work. The workbook will present strategies for you to try and help you understand how to make changes. But, as with all self-help books, you must help yourself.

So before you continue reading this book, look over the following statements and check the one that applies to you now. Be honest with yourself. Don't check the statement that you think you should check, or the statement that you think others would want you to check. If you start with an honest assessment of your readiness to change, you can avoid setting yourself up for failure and can gain the maximum value from this workbook.

- [ ] 1. Right now, I am ready and willing to work hard to learn to manage my irritable bowel.
- [ ] 2. I would like to manage my irritable bowel better, but I am not sure how hard I am able to work to learn new things right now.
- [ ] 3. I am thinking about making changes to better manage my irritable bowel, but the timing is not great right now.
- [ ] 4. This is not a good time for me to work on my irritable bowel. I may be more able sometime in the future.

If you checked statement 1, you are ready to take action to manage your irritable bowel; this workbook is ideal for you. In addition to providing you with information, it will mostly guide you through hands-on techniques that will allow you to determine the pattern of your symptoms, identify the things that trigger your symptoms, and, based on this, take action to control your symptoms. We cover a lot of material in this workbook, so go slowly. You might find it useful to read a chapter once to get an idea of the scope of topics covered and the range of things that you will be asked to do. Then read the chapter again, going slowly and practicing the strategies presented. Also, we present the techniques used in this workbook in what we call a "cafeteria" approach. By this we mean that you should feel free to pick and choose specific methods that feel right and work for you. This will allow you to match the method to your symptoms, personality, and lifestyle.

If you checked statement 2, you are preparing for change but might not actually be ready to change right now. You should find this workbook helpful in providing information and giving you some ideas about how to change. We recommend that you try the methods we suggest, but don't be surprised if you're not fully prepared to put all the effort and commitment to following through with them. Try them as a way of helping you decide on the costs and benefits of this workbook. If after you have gone through the workbook you decide you are ready to commit yourself, it may be helpful to read the workbook again to gain maximum value from the techniques.

If you checked statement 3, you are only thinking about change but are not ready to commit yourself. This workbook will be useful as a source of information and as a reference if you decide that you do want to try to change. Don't expect big results from anything you try if you checked this box. For the workbook to make a significant impact on your symptoms, you've got to be willing to keep using the methods; this requires an upfront commitment. If you're not ready for this commitment, you're just not ready. Don't beat yourself up for this. It may help if you write a list of the advantages and disadvantages of using this workbook, and a list of the negatives of having irritable bowel. Only when people experience significant distress about having irritable bowel and see more advantages than disadvantages in trying to control symptoms through healthy eating and stress management are they able to commit energy and effort into a workbook like this.

If you checked statement 4, it is likely that someone else has suggested you read this book. You may be doing it for that person and not for yourself. If this is you, don't expect much from this workbook. The most you will get out of this book is information that may help you decide to change at some point in the future.

We wrote this book to accomplish two goals. First, we want to help you determine if your symptoms actually fit those of irritable bowel. Chapters 1 and 2, in particular, cover the diagnosis of irritable bowel. If your symptoms do not point to irritable bowel, you should see your doctor to check for the presence of a bowel disease such as Crohn's disease or ulcerative colitis. Second, this book will teach you a better way of living with your particular irritable bowel symptoms. We will outline detailed changes that you can make to your eating habits and provide you with stress management techniques.

As you read this book, be advised: *don't expect a cure*. We will help you to manage your symptoms and limit the frequency, intensity, and duration of irritable bowel episodes. Still, irritable bowel tends to be chronic and is related to the way that your bowel is put together. Irritable bowel often goes through episodes of good and bad functioning. Also, stress and eating patterns fluctuate, and for some people these factors routinely bring on symptoms.

This is not meant to be bad news. Instead, it is meant to help you develop realistic expectations for this book and, for that matter, any treatment for irritable bowel. Our patients tell us that they don't need a cure (though none would refuse one if it were available). They say it is sufficient to be in control of their bowel rather than to feel, as many do before they attend our clinic, that their bowel is in control of them.

1

What Is IBS?

At the outset, we want to clear up some terminology issues. IBS is the abbreviation that doctors use for irritable bowel syndrome, often when they are talking about people with IBS. We will *not* be using the term IBS in this book; instead, we will use the less confusing label *irritable bowel* for this disorder.

Why not use IBS? We have found that abbreviations can cause confusion between diseases and medical conditions. For instance, IBS (irritable bowel syndrome) is often confused with IBD (inflammatory bowel disease). By changing one letter, you go from having a condition (irritable bowel) that causes no serious medical complications to having a disease (inflammatory bowel) that includes serious bowel diseases such as Crohn's disease and ulcerative colitis. Using the term *irritable bowel* avoids this confusion.

We also dislike using IBS because the term *syndrome* is easily misunderstood. *Syndrome* can have a negative connotation, and it is often associated with mental problems or conditions. *Syndrome* actually refers to a collection of symptoms that helps diagnose certain medical (and mental) conditions. We don't like the word, however, and neither do our patients, so we will not use it again in this book.

Another confusing term that has been used to describe irritable bowel is *mucous colitis*. Thankfully, few doctors still use this term, but we feel it should be banished altogether. It frequently causes people to focus on the colitis label and think they have a serious bowel disease. As you will learn, mucus in the stool is a common symptom of irritable bowel, but colitis is a medical term implying that the large bowel or colon is inflamed. There is no significant inflammation of the bowel with irritable bowel (see chapter 4), even though some of the symptoms, such as diarrhea and abdominal pain, may mimic those associated with inflammation.

Diagnosing Irritable Bowel

Irritable bowel is diagnosed by its symptoms, not by a particular medical test. That's because irritable bowel is a normal, healthy bowel, both to the naked eye and under the microscope. For some reason, though, irritable bowel does not coordinate its functions normally. It is also extra-sensitive to food, stress, and other stimulants. However, irritable bowel does *not* lead to bowel cancer or other serious bowel diseases such as colitis, Crohn's disease, or ulcers. (See chapter 3 for information on how the bowel and the entire digestive tract normally work and the problems that can occur with irritable bowel.)

Doctors look for a specific pattern of symptoms when diagnosing irritable bowel. If you have had at least three of the six most common symptoms for more than three months—without symptoms that might indicate bowel disease (see chapter 2)—then you meet the criteria for a diagnosis of irritable bowel. The more symptoms you experience, the more likely it is that you have irritable bowel.

Symptoms of Irritable Bowel

Symptoms include:

- Abdominal pain for at least three months. It can be present continuously, but more often it is intermittent (on and off over time). The pain is relieved with a bowel movement.
- Increased frequency of bowel movements when the pain occurs. Alternatively, infrequent bowel movements (constipation) may be experienced at other times.

- Increased looseness of the stool when the abdominal pain is felt. At other times, the stool form may be hard or constipated.
- Mucus in the stool.
- A sensation of incomplete emptying of the rectum after going to the bathroom.
- A bloated or distended feeling in the abdomen.

To rule out serious disease, doctors usually perform a physical examination, along with a few simple blood tests. Experienced doctors need few tests to diagnose irritable bowel, especially when at least three of the symptoms listed are present and there are no unusual or worrisome symptoms. Although distressing at times, irritable bowel symptoms do not mean there is anything wrong with the intestine. Even if the symptoms are frequent and severe, it does not mean that anything harmful will happen or develop in the bowel.

Symptoms *Not* Related to Irritable Bowel

The most important symptom to watch for is blood in the stool. Bleeding does not occur with irritable bowel. If you see blood in your stool, you need to see your doctor. The bleeding may or may not signal a serious disease, but it is not an irritable bowel symptom, which is why you should talk to your doctor.

Do your bowel symptoms cause you to wake from sleep? If so, this is very unusual with irritable bowel. Bowel symptoms arise from bowel activity, and your bowel goes to sleep when you do. Although waking from sleep with bowel symptoms and pain can occur at times, this usually indicates an underlying disease of the bowel.

Finally, fever and unexplained weight loss are not related to irritable bowel, so we urge you to see your doctor if you have these symptoms.

Does Irritable Bowel Cause Other Problems?

People with irritable bowel can have a number of other symptoms in other parts of the body. The following symptoms cannot be used to diagnose irritable bowel, but they are commonly associated with it:

- *Urinary problems* are quite common and usually involve feeling the need to pass urine more frequently, often with urgency.

- *Migraine headaches* occur more often in people with irritable bowel than in people without it.
- *Painful sexual intercourse* for women, presumably because the surrounding pelvic structures, such as the bladder and the bowel, are also oversensitive or "irritable."
- *Fatigue* is very common. Generally, its source is unclear, but in context with the common symptoms of irritable bowel, fatigue often can be linked with this condition.
- *Heartburn* is also frequently experienced by people with irritable bowel. This may reflect the increased bowel sensitivity, which can affect the esophagus and the stomach and cause heartburn or indigestion. There are many other causes for heartburn and indigestion, however, so you should see your doctor if you suffer mostly with these symptoms.
- *Fibromyalgia*, a poorly understood disorder that causes chronic muscle pain, fatigue, memory problems, and other symptoms, is found more commonly in people with irritable bowel.

Who Experiences Irritable Bowel?

Research studies over the last twenty years have led to a much better understanding of irritable bowel. We now know, for instance, that irritable bowel usually strikes young, healthy adults. Many people start to experience symptoms before they turn thirty. In fact, if you are over forty and are suddenly having irritable bowel symptoms for the first time, you should see your doctor. A recent intestinal infection could be the culprit. Research shows that an infection that causes inflammation of the bowel can result in a prolonged disturbance in bowel control even after the inflammation heals and the offending organism is cleared from the body. In most people, bowel function gradually returns to normal.

As mentioned earlier, irritable bowel symptoms arise from disordered coordination of the bowel and because the bowel is more sensitive than normal. An estimated 10 to 15 percent of the population in North America have irritable bowel. Actually, with so much activity in the gut during and between meals, it is surprising that irritable bowel isn't more prevalent. Most people appear to be completely oblivious to intestinal activity. Even so, irritable bowel is the second leading cause of absenteeism from work and school behind the common cold.

All told, irritable bowel affects twice as many women as men, particularly in Western cultures such as North America and western Europe. Studies around the globe find people with irritable bowel in parts of Africa, China, India, and other countries. Interestingly, in India more men than women report symptoms, though we do not know why this occurs in India and not elsewhere.

Irritable bowel symptoms do not occur persistently in an individual. They appear to come and go over time, often triggered or worsened by dietary factors and stress. About half of the population with irritable bowel seeks medical attention. Not surprisingly, a visit to the doctor usually depends on the frequency and severity of symptoms.

Men and women generally experience the same symptoms, though abdominal bloating is more common in women. Both men and women see doctors if they have a lot of abdominal pain or multiple bowel symptoms. However, men are more likely to seek medical attention if they are having frequent bouts of diarrhea.

For anyone, the fear of losing control of the bowel can be very disabling and stressful. Sometimes diarrhea and the urgency to pass stool can be so intense that it causes incontinence or loss of bowel control. If you have this problem, you should see your doctor. Many treatments are available to control fecal incontinence, especially if the incontinence is with loose, watery stools.

If You've Been Told Your Symptoms Are "All in Your Head"

Irritable bowel symptoms are real. They occur because the bowel is not working in a normal, coordinated manner. Unfortunately, many doctors lead patients to believe that because no abnormalities can be found on either X-rays or blood tests their symptoms must be "in their head." This is incorrect. It is our intention to dispel the myth.

Understanding that the intestines are more sensitive than other organs may actually serve as a useful guide for you to help monitor other aspects of your life. What will follow in subsequent chapters is a discussion of how you can use the symptoms of irritable bowel to adjust your diet and to evaluate the effects of stress on your body. Irritable bowel may actually serve as an early warning system: when you are eating a diet that is not ideal for your body (for example, high fat or high caffeine intake), your gut will let you know it doesn't like these foods. Perhaps even more important, a sensitive gut may help you to identify when you are experiencing stress in certain situations or from life events because of the increase in your intestinal symptoms. Adjusting what you are doing when you experience irritable bowel symptoms may help to minimize or alleviate the stressful conditions in a more positive and healthy manner. You will learn more about these techniques when you read about diet in chapters 5, 6, and 7 and the effects of stress on irritable bowel in chapter 8.

It's not uncommon for patients to look to medications or over-the-counter preparations such as laxatives to relieve their symptoms. Unfortunately, long-term and frequent use of these drugs can actually damage the gut and aggravate problems. That's why it is best to avoid relying on drugs to manage your symptoms and to instead learn the techniques in this book.

No single drug will treat all the symptoms of irritable bowel, and any attempt to develop such a drug would probably be unsuccessful. The majority of people with irritable bowel experience symptoms off and on throughout their lives. It would not make sense for these healthy individuals to take drugs for thirty or forty years, especially when potential side effects and long-term effects are difficult to predict.

Take a few moments now to complete the following questionnaire. This questionnaire will help you identify your irritable bowel symptoms and help you begin to link symptoms to treatment. Chapter 2 will elaborate on some of the concepts we have discussed and help you to confirm if you do indeed have irritable bowel.

Do I Have Irritable Bowel?

For each question, check the answer that applies. At the end of the questionnaire, score your answers to see if you have irritable bowel.

		Yes	No
1.	In the past three months have you had continuous or repeated discomfort or pain in your lower abdomen? (If no, skip to question 5.)	☑	☐
2.	Is this discomfort or pain relieved by a bowel movement?	☑	☐
3.	Is this discomfort or pain associated with a change in the frequency of bowel movements (for example, having more or fewer bowel movements)?	☐	☐
4.	Is this discomfort or pain associated with a change in the consistency of the stool (for example, softer or harder)?	☑	☐

5. Would you say that on at least one-fourth of the days in the last three months you have had any of the following (check all that apply):

   ☐ Fewer than three bowel movements a week

   ☐ More than three bowel movements a day

   ☐ Hard or lumpy stools

   ☐ Loose or watery stools

   ☐ Straining during a bowel movement

   ☐ Urgency—having to rush to the bathroom for a bowel movement

   ☐ Feeling of incomplete emptying after a bowel movement

   ☐ Passing mucus (whitish substance) during a bowel movement

   ☐ Abdominal fullness, bloating, or swelling

		Yes	No
6.	If you have had loose or watery stools, would you say that they occurred with more than three-fourths of your total bowel movements in the past three months?	☑	☐
7.	If you have had over three bowel movements a day, would you say that this occurred on more than half of the days in the past three months?	☑	☐
8.	In the past three months, have you noticed a large amount of stool when you go to the bathroom?	☐	☐

Yes No

9. Over the past six months, have you had continuous or frequently recurring pain in your abdomen? (If you are female, this should not be related to your menstrual cycle or period.) (If no, skip to question 11.)   ☐ ☐

10. Has this pain interfered with your daily activities from time to time (for example, an inability to work or a decrease in social events)?   ☐ ☐

11. Do you suffer from frequent headaches, or has your doctor told you that you have migraine headaches?   ☐ ☐

12. Do you suffer from fatigue or feel very tired most days to the point that it interferes with your daily activities such as being able to work or take part in social activities?   ☐ ☐

13. Do you suffer from recurrent muscle and joint aches or pains or has your doctor told you that you have a condition called fibromyalgia?   ☐ ☐

14. If you are female, in the past three months have you suffered from discomfort or pain during sexual intercourse?   ☐ ☐

15. In the past three months have you had to rush to the bathroom to pass urine, or do you often feel that you have to pass urine while up during the day?   ☐ ☐

16. Do you ever see blood in your bowel movements?   ☐ ☐

17. Do you wake from a deep sleep at night with your bowel symptoms or with abdominal discomfort or pain?   ☐ ☐

18. When you are troubled by your bowel symptoms, do you ever experience fever (that is, a temperature greater than 100°F)?   ☐ ☐

19. In the past three months have you noticed weight loss without attempting to restrict or change your diet?   ☐ ☐

20. Do you vomit when you have abdominal discomfort or pain?   ☐ ☐

21. If you answered yes to any of questions 1 through 9, are you over forty years old and experiencing these symptoms for the first time ever in your life?   ☐ ☐

If you answered yes to questions 1 and 2 or 3 or 4 and you checked two or more responses to question 5, then you have irritable bowel.

If you answered yes on question 5, to the first, third, fifth, and/or seventh items, then you have constipation-predominant irritable bowel and you should consider increasing dietary fiber and fluid in your diet. (See the high-fiber diet in chapter 7.)

If you answered yes to questions 6, 7, and/or 8, then you have diarrhea-predominant irritable bowel and you may not find increasing dietary fiber especially helpful. If you wish to try adding more fiber to your diet, you should introduce the fiber very gradually because it could make your diarrhea worse. Other possible diet adjustments are important to explore because certain foods and beverages can worsen diarrhea (see chapter 7).

If you answered yes to question 5, item 9, then you have problems with abdominal bloating (see chapter 7).

You may have a more serious bowel disorder if you answered yes to any of questions 16 through 21. If you answered yes to any of these questions, you should see your doctor.

If you answered yes to questions 9 and 10, then you have a significant problem with abdominal pain. People with predominant abdominal pain without a direct connection to bowel function may have a disorder called *chronic functional abdominal pain*, which in some people may be linked to a past history of physical, sexual, or emotional abuse. People with these past events will need special therapy and should talk to their doctors about seeing a therapist with expertise in these areas. (See chapter 10 for additional information about dealing with pain if it is your primary complaint.)

If you answered yes to questions 11 through 15, then you have some of the common nonbowel symptoms associated with irritable bowel. These symptoms can all be treated by your doctor, and you may also find this book helpful since improving the bowel symptoms of irritable bowel often helps decrease the severity of the associated nonbowel symptoms.

2

How Do I Know I Have Irritable Bowel?

As you now know, medical tests cannot determine whether or not you have irritable bowel. Tests can only exclude other diseases that might cause your symptoms. Instead, it is the particular symptoms that you experience that determine whether you are diagnosed with irritable bowel. In this chapter, we will spend more time explaining and reviewing some of the concepts already introduced. We will also provide more information about how a diagnosis is actually made.

Pain: The Number-One Symptom

It can be frightening and confusing to experience the symptoms of irritable bowel—especially if the symptoms are painful. All of us have learned to avoid pain from our earliest years, and most of us automatically interpret pain as a signal that something must be wrong. Unfortunately, recurring bouts of abdominal pain for at least three months is the main symptom of irritable bowel. It is also the most common reason to seek a doctor's advice. Pain does not always mean there is a serious disease, however. This is especially true with irritable bowel.

The pain associated with irritable bowel is often located in the lower part of the abdomen below the belly button, but it can be felt throughout the abdomen. The pain occurs because of the bowel's heightened sensitivity (see chapter 4). After a bowel movement, the bowel relaxes and the pain usually goes away, often returning a few minutes later. This is quite characteristic of irritable bowel and is less commonly seen with bowel diseases. If there is a serious disease such as colitis or inflammation of the bowel, the pain often lingers though the intensity may decrease. This is because the pain is due to the inflammation of the bowel, which continues even though the contractions to cause a bowel movement have stopped.

Although pain is normal with irritable bowel, it does not mean you cannot or should not do anything about it. Changing your eating habits and practicing stress management techniques (explained later in this book) will help ease your symptoms, as will following the advice in chapter 10, which details the best ways to manage pain. Still, you shouldn't hesitate to see your doctor about abdominal pain, especially if it has surfaced recently, is very severe, or you have never experienced a similar pain.

The Other Diagnostic Symptoms

When you are experiencing abdominal pain, you may notice that there is a change in your stool pattern. Bowel movements occur more frequently, usually becoming liquid and watery. A typical pattern is the onset of abdominal pain, with a temporary relief of pain after a somewhat formed bowel movement. This is followed by repeated spasms of pain, with increasingly looser bowel movements (more and more liquid in the stool). The pain and the frequent trips to the bathroom often occur over several hours, leaving many people feeling drained and exhausted.

Another common symptom of irritable bowel is an irregular pattern of bowel movements occurring at least 25 percent of the time. For instance, you might have a regular bowel movement every day, but every fourth week your bowel movements are either more constipated or looser and diarrhealike. In fact, having isolated episodes of irregular bowel function—interspersed with normal bowel function—is more typical of irritable bowel than of bowel diseases. When the bowel is inflamed, which occurs with Crohn's disease, colitis, and other bowel diseases, the change in bowel habits usually lasts several weeks until the inflammation settles. This bowel movement pattern distinguishes irritable bowel symptoms from more serious bowel diseases.

The presence of mucus in the stool is another symptom of irritable bowel. Many people believe that mucus in the stool indicates that they have a serious bowel disease, such as colitis. In fact, mucus alone (without blood) is a common finding in irritable bowel patients, but not in patients with colitis. People with colitis see blood mixed with the mucus in the stool.

Mucus, which is produced by the intestines, is a normal product of the bowel and serves as a lubricant. A symptom of irritable bowel is the production of more mucus than necessary. Mucus is particularly visible if the stool is loose, but it can also appear in a constipated bowel motion. On occasion, patients may even pass mucus alone without stool.

Another common symptom of irritable bowel, especially if you are constipated, is abdominal bloating or swelling. The bloating, which can often be quite pronounced, is usually worse later in the day and after eating. It frequently disappears or improves significantly overnight during sleep but then recurs the following day. Bloating that varies throughout the course of the day is seen only with irritable bowel. Serious conditions such as a fluid collection in the abdomen or a tumor growth will cause abdominal swelling, but they do not come and go over a twenty-four-hour period.

Finally, the sixth common symptom of irritable bowel is a sensation of incomplete emptying of the rectum after a bowel movement. This often causes a great deal of distress and concern. People frequently feel that their bowel motions are incomplete, and they strain excessively to try to pass stool. This symptom again reflects the irritability or, perhaps more appropriately, the increased sensitivity of the gut. In most people with this symptom, the rectum has indeed emptied completely, and the feeling of incomplete emptying is a false sensation caused by an oversensitive rectum.

Other Symptoms Associated
with Irritable Bowel

As mentioned in chapter 1, symptoms in parts of the body other than the intestines can often accompany irritable bowel. Several studies show that symptoms of heartburn occur more often in people with irritable bowel than in those without it. Heartburn involves the stomach and the esophagus, while irritable bowel involves the intestines. The occurrence of irritable bowel and heartburn together might indicate that the whole digestive system is more sensitive than usual.

Another common nonbowel symptom for people with irritable bowel is fatigue. Recent studies show that many people with severe irritable bowel symptoms have disturbed sleep patterns, and this disruption may further aggravate or accentuate a tendency to have irritable bowel symptoms. Fatigue may also point to more serious psychological problems such as depression (see chapter 12). Sometimes irritable bowel symptoms will improve as sleep patterns are restored. Irritable bowel symptoms always improve if depression is treated.

Bladder or urinary problems are also associated with irritable bowel. There may be times when you feel you have to pass urine more frequently, or you may experience a sudden urge to pass urine. You may even feel as though you are about to lose control. Yet when you actually urinate, there may not be much urine at all. The source of this sensation is unknown; however, it may be that there is a generalized sensitivity in the smooth muscle, which lines the bowel and the bladder. Smooth muscle sensitivity could explain why migraine headaches are linked to irritable bowel. Smooth muscle lines the intestines and also lines the blood vessels that cause the throbbing effect of migraine headaches. Still, the factors that lead to migraine headaches are much more complicated, and at present it is unclear why migraine headaches and irritable bowel occur together.

It's common for women to notice that their irritable bowel symptoms appear around the time of their menstrual cycle. If this happens to you, try your best to avoid any other triggers that can bring on or worsen bowel symptoms, such as certain foods and stress or anxiety. The combination of these triggers will increase the intensity of your symptoms during your period. Painful intercourse can often trouble women with irritable bowel symptoms. Sensitive organs in the pelvis, including the bladder and the bowel, may contribute to this pain.

Some people with irritable bowel also suffer from a condition called *fibromyalgia*. This condition could be called *irritable bowel of the muscles*. In this condition, for unknown reasons, the muscles and the tendons are more sensitive and have areas of localized tenderness and pain. Again, pain is the major symptom, and it can aggravate irritable bowel symptoms. Fibromyalgia can aggravate irritable bowel symptoms because of pain in the muscles in the abdominal wall. Abdominal pain can be quite intense and persistent because the abdominal wall muscles are large, powerful muscles that we use all day (as we do our back muscles). When they become sensitive and prone to pain, achieving pain relief can be difficult. Abdominal muscles are called *postural muscles* because they are used to support the body and maintain posture. We use these muscles even when we are sitting in a chair or lying down. Even shifting your weight to roll onto your side may trigger pain. Because of all these factors, abdominal pain can be persistent and keep relapsing. Chapter 10 covers pain management techniques.

Pinpointing Your Symptoms

As you explore whether irritable bowel is indeed the reason for the symptoms you are experiencing, it will help to complete the checklist on page 20 before your next doctor's visit. Irritable bowel can usually be diagnosed without a lot of tests. However, common symptoms of irritable bowel can mimic or overlap those of other bowel conditions or diseases.

If you have any concerns or do not feel that your symptoms exactly fit those of irritable bowel, then you should seek the advice of your doctor. Not only will the checklist help to determine whether you meet the criteria for irritable bowel, but it will also serve as an up-to-date list of your symptoms.

Symptom List

Show your doctor this list.

		Yes	No
1.	Pain in the lower half of the belly or abdomen.	☑	☐
2.	Pain present for ____ weeks.	☑	☐
3.	Abdominal pain is relieved when I have a bowel motion.	☑	☐
4.	Bowel movements are looser when I have the pain.	☒	☐
5.	I have more frequent bowel motions with the pain.	☒	☐
6.	I am constipated when I have the pain.	☒	☐
7.	I have to strain to make my bowels work.	☑	☐
8.	I have to rush to the bathroom for fear of losing control of my bowels.	☒	☐
9.	I feel I don't finish when I do have a bowel motion.	☒	☐
10.	I see mucus (slime) when I have a bowel motion.	☐	☐
11.	I feel bloated and have swelling of my belly.	☒	☐
12.	I feel tired all the time.	☒	☐
13.	I have frequent headaches.	☒	☐
14.	I frequently have muscle and joint aches.	☒	☐
15.	I have to rush to the bathroom when I pass urine.	☒	☐
16.	I have trouble sleeping.	☒	☐

Bowel Symptoms I *Must* Tell My Doctor About

		Yes	No
1.	I see blood in my stool or bowel motions.	☐	☐
2.	I see black bowel motions.	☐	☐
3.	I have noted a fever. My temperature was: _____.	☐	☐
4.	I have been noticing weight loss without being on a weight-reducing diet. I have lost _____ lbs. in the past _____ months.	☐	☐
5.	I have noticed the pain can wake me out of a deep sleep at night.	☐	☐
6.	The pain causes me to vomit.	☐	☐
7.	I have seen blood or black-colored material when I have vomited.	☐	☐

Making It Fit: Identifying Your Symptoms and Patterns of Functioning

For this book to be useful, you need to see improvements in your own symptoms. It is not enough for us to talk about general issues concerning irritable bowel, diet, and stress. We want to help you identify the specific symptoms that you experience and their connections to eating, stress, and other factors.

In our clinical work, this is straightforward; we simply ask questions and receive answers from our patients about their symptoms and their circumstances. We cannot do this in a book. You must assess yourself.

One of the best ways to monitor and identify your symptoms is to complete over a one-week period the diary at the end of this chapter. The information you collect during the week will help you become familiar with the specifics of your symptoms, and you will begin to discover connections between your diet, stress, and symptoms. These insights will be particularly helpful as you read the chapters on healthy eating and stress.

Recording unpleasant symptoms for a week may seem like a long time when you want relief, but we find that it takes at least a week to identify patterns of stress, eating, and symptoms. The connection among stress, eating, and symptoms is not necessarily immediate and clear. Stress that occurs one day may not affect the bowel for several days. Furthermore, it may not affect the bowel to the same degree, and in the same way, each time. General feelings and worries can also influence how you experience your bowel symptoms. If you are worried that your symptoms are due to cancer, your symptoms will cause more alarm than if you realize they are due to a slice of pizza you ate.

A symptoms diary is necessary because you need to be able to collect enough information so you can stand back and observe patterns. Often, we have patients who can't see the forest for the trees. They tell us, "I was really stressed Tuesday at work, but my bowel was fine. On Thursday I couldn't stand the pain, but everything was calm—I had no stress." Similar delayed patterns occur for eating as well.

We want to emphasize the importance of self-assessment. Successfully managing irritable bowel symptoms requires matching management strategies to symptoms and understanding the links among stress, eating, and symptoms that are specific to you. All individuals are unique. Plus, while we have expertise in the medical, nutritional, and psychological aspects of irritable bowel, you are the expert on you.

In the chapters that follow, we will ask you to refer to your symptoms diary. This will make it much easier for you to choose the best strategies. We will ask you to fill out a diary again after you have worked through the exercises in the upcoming chapters. This will allow you to evaluate how successful the program has been and allow you to compare yourself from before to after.

To complete the diary, first choose a time each day to fill it out. Many people prefer the end of the day, when they can think more clearly and can review the day's events while they are still fresh in their minds. Each time you complete the diary, write down the date and time. Then record any irritable bowel symptoms you experienced that day and their severity. Try to summarize each symptom in one or two words using the symptom list on pages 6 and 7. Beside each symptom, write the number that corresponds to the severity of the symptom. Use a rating between 1 and 10, where 1 means not at all severe, 5 means moderately severe, and 10 means extremely severe.

Next, consider what you ate. Try to identify any foods or patterns of eating that you suspect might have triggered your symptoms. Did you eat anything that might have upset you? Did you skip any meals or eat too fast?

It's not easy to identify possible food-related triggers, so don't worry if you have trouble at this point. The chapters on nutrition and stress will help you learn how to pinpoint foods that may be a problem for you. Right now, we simply want you to start thinking about possible triggers. Jot down anything that you suspect is a food trigger. Otherwise, make a brief note about what you ate.

Next, rate your daily stress level using a scale of 1 to 10 (1 for not at all stressed, 5 for moderately stressed, and 10 for extremely stressed). If you were stressed, make a brief note about the source of the stress.

Sometimes people become so accustomed to stress that they have trouble identifying it. Don't worry if this is the case. Just ask yourself: What was stressful about today? Again, at this stage we just want to help you begin to identify patterns.

Finally, we want you to identify any feelings and worries that relate to your symptoms of irritable bowel. In the last row of the table, write down the feelings that are associated with your symptoms, such as anxiety, frustration, or sadness. Also, if you are aware of any worrisome thoughts, write them here. This will help you to determine how your thoughts and concerns affect the severity or onset of your symptoms.

Do your best to complete the symptoms diary each day. It may seem awkward at first, but after two or three days, you will get the hang of it. Almost everyone who completes a diary for a whole week learns something important about their irritable bowel.

SYMPTOMS DIARY

	Symptoms (note time as well)	Severity of Symptoms (1 = minimal/negligible; 10 = extreme severity)	Food Triggers (that is, foods eaten *before* symptoms)	Stress Level (1 = no stress; 10 = extreme stress)	Feelings and Worries
Monday					
Tuesday					
Wednesday					

	Symptoms (note time as well)	Severity of Symptoms (1 = minimal/negligible; 10 = extreme severity)	Food Triggers (that is, foods eaten before symptoms)	Stress Level (1 = no stress; 10 = extreme stress)	Feelings and Worries
Thursday					
Friday					
Saturday					
Sunday					

25

3

How the Gut Works, and Sometimes Doesn't

The digestive tract is an often overlooked and underappreciated part of the body. Usually, we rank the brain or the heart higher on the list of importance. The gut is vital for the nutritional support of the body, however, and it plays a crucial role in our overall health. The symptoms of irritable bowel mostly result from problems that originate in the large intestine or the colon, though recent research indicates that irritable bowel can disrupt the entire gut.

The word *gut* refers to several digestive organs, including the intestines (bowels), the stomach, and the esophagus, as well as the pancreas and the bile system (see figures 1, 2, and 3 later in this chapter). The gut is organized into three parts—esophagus, stomach, and intestines—and it serves several purposes. It is designed to take in nourishment and then process it so that the body can absorb and use the food we eat. The gut also provides an *infection barrier* between the environment outside the body (where our food comes from) and the inside of our bodies. In addition, the gut helps our bodies to maximize their fluid and calorie sources by absorbing fluid from our food and regulating the materials that leave our bodies as waste.

The Esophagus

The esophagus is essentially a pipe that transmits food from the mouth to the stomach. Digestion actually begins in the mouth. Special products that the body uses to break down food, known as *enzymes*, are released in the mouth. The enzymes in the mouth help to break down starchy foods. If you have ever chewed a plain cracker or a piece of bread slowly, you might have noticed it begin to taste sweeter. This is because the enzymes in your saliva turn complex carbohydrates (the starch in flour) into simple carbohydrates, which taste sweet to us. Saliva also helps to lubricate food, and chewing breaks the food into smaller chunks, making it easier for the food to pass down the esophagus into the stomach.

Esophageal Problems in Irritable Bowel

Acid causes a sensation of *heartburn* if it gets back into the esophagus, and this sometimes occurs in people with irritable bowel. There is a muscle valve, or *sphincter*, at the lower end of the esophagus that contracts in between swallows to keep food and stomach acid in the stomach and out of the esophagus. A weak *lower esophageal sphincter* (LES) can allow acid into the esophagus, damaging the esophageal lining and causing pain. A weak LES and esophageal muscle also have a hard time pushing acid (or food) back into the stomach. Episodes of chest pain can feel like heart pain, but if a doctor rules out heart pain, then a sensitive esophageal lining and/or spasms in the esophagus can also cause chest pain. Emotional stress can bring on spasms and pain in the esophagus or aggravate existing pain. Certain foods (and liquids) can also trigger these abnormal muscle contractions and activate chemical sensors in the lining of the esophagus to produce pain. In other words, the normal gut activity of taking in food or liquid triggers pain, which is a common theme in the mechanisms of symptom generation in irritable bowel (see chapter 4).

The Stomach

Food travels down the esophagus to the stomach, taking only seconds or, at most, a few minutes. In the stomach, churning and stomach acid break down the food into a more digestible liquid mush. Stomach acid is important in preparing the protein in foods we eat for digestion in the small intestine. Though stomach acid helps break down food particles, especially proteins, it is not required to digest food. We know this because individuals can live without a stomach while maintaining their nutritional status. Others live with a stomach that is unable to produce acid and also have no problems digesting food. However, without stomach acid people are much more likely to get an intestinal infection since stomach acid kills harmful organisms such as bacteria, parasites, and viruses. In addition, acid in the stomach helps us to absorb iron from vegetables and grains, but not from meats. The iron in meats is readily absorbed by the small intestine without help from stomach acid. The acid-producing cells in the stomach also produce a factor needed for vitamin B_{12} absorption in the small intestine.

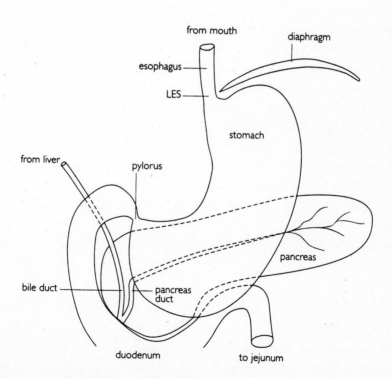

Figure 1   The upper gastrointestinal tract

Stomach Problems in Irritable Bowel

Perhaps the stomach's most essential function is to serve as a reservoir for food, allowing us to eat large quantities of food intermittently. Irritable bowel can cause this reservoir function of the stomach to not work as well. Eating large meals, particularly meals of fatty foods that empty more slowly from the stomach anyway, can produce a feeling of abdominal distension in irritable bowel. Just like the esophagus, the stomach can be sensitive to distension, and even normal-sized meals can produce pain and discomfort in irritable bowel. Because the stomach is sensitive in irritable bowel, meals have to be eaten regularly because the stomach doesn't like to be bloated with food. If you go for too long between meals, stomach acid will be more likely to produce symptoms in your sensitive gut and can also trigger air swallowing that contributes to bloating.

Air swallowing is common and often occurs when people are under stress or have a bloated full feeling. Often without realizing they are doing it, they will swallow, which causes air to be moved down the esophagus, with the swallow, into the stomach. This then triggers burping to bring the air up to relieve the bloated feeling. Unfortunately, if you have an irritable bowel, this causes not only burping but also more air in the gut, which increases the bloated feeling and does not relieve the bloating. Poor gas handling in irritable bowel is further discussed later in this chapter.

Emptying of the stomach can also be delayed in irritable bowel, and again, this delay is more likely if you have eaten fatty foods. When the stomach stays full for a long time, it is easier for stomach acid to regurgitate back into the esophagus, especially if the stomach is overstretched with food. Furthermore, fatty foods release a hormone when they are digested in the small intestine that further relaxes the LES between the muscle and the esophagus, further contributing to acid reflux and heartburn.

The Intestine

Once the stomach has churned food into a liquid pulp, small quantities are gradually released through a special muscle valve opening between the stomach and the small intestine called the *pylorus*. Food that comes through the pylorus enters the beginning of the small intestine known as the *duodenum*. The pancreas and the bile duct empty into this part of the small intestine, releasing bicarbonate products that neutralize the stomach acid mixed with the food. Besides bicarbonates, the bile and the pancreatic secretions are extremely important in the digestion of food.

Bile is made in the liver and stored in the gallbladder until it is released into the small intestine. Bile plays a key role in digesting fat, which is the most difficult foodstuff for the small intestine to break down and absorb. A number of hormones are released into the bloodstream from the duodenum when fat comes into contact with the duodenal lining. These hormones tell the pancreas to release its digestive juices and the gallbladder to release bile into the duodenum. The release of these products causes the small intestine to begin its pattern of muscle contraction that helps the gut to digest the food as well as to maximize the absorption of nutrients into the body.

Bile adds large quantities of fluid and salts or *electrolytes* to the food, keeping it in a liquid state. As food moves through the small intestine, enzymes from the pancreas and the small intestine itself break it down further. In the presence of bile salts (which break the fat globules into smaller more soluble globules called *micelles*), the enzymes from the pancreas can digest the fat so that the body can absorb it. The food that is absorbed from the small intestine enters the bloodstream and is transported to the liver, which cleanses the blood and sends the nutrients into the bloodstream. The nutrients then flow to the rest of the body, providing what the cells need for their metabolism and function.

Given the number of digestive functions that the small intestine performs, it is clearly a vital organ for life. The small intestine also has a huge surface area, estimated at the size of a football field. Because there is so much surface area, there is always close contact between the food and the cells lining the small intestine, maximizing the absorption of the component parts of food. Essentially, food can be broken down into four components:

1. Carbohydrates are broken down into sugars.
2. Proteins are broken down into amino acids.
3. Fat is broken down into fatty acids and glycerol.
4. Specific vitamins and minerals that are necessary for health are extracted from foods.

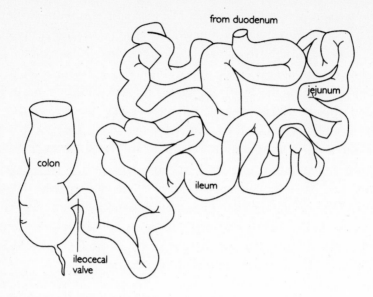

from duodenum

jejunum

colon

ileum

ileocecal
valve

Figure 2   The small intestine

Small Intestine Problems in Irritable Bowel

People with irritable bowel also have a sensitive small intestine. Most people do not feel the frequent contractions of the small intestine, but with irritable bowel, sometimes even normal contractions can produce pain or discomfort. Gas can also be a problem. Even though irritable bowel may not produce more gas, a normal amount of gas in the intestines that would give someone with a "normal" bowel no problems can cause bloating and distension in people with irritable bowel. Irritable bowel can also make it more difficult for the gut to move gas through the intestines to be expelled. These problems with handling gas are believed to cause the bloating symptom often experienced by irritable bowel sufferers.

Diarrhea-predominant irritable bowel may be due to less bile salt absorption in the last part of the small intestine (ileum) in some people. Bile salts act like a laxative if they enter the colon, so if you don't absorb them normally in the ileum, they can trigger diarrhea. People who have had their gallbladders removed frequently experience diarrhea because more bile salts get into the colon when the gallbladder is removed. If you already have irritable bowel, having your gallbladder removed will often worsen your symptoms because of this tendency to experience diarrhea after surgery. If your gallbladder is diseased, however, it will need to be removed; there are medications that will help control the loss of bile salts into the colon to reduce or eliminate the diarrhea.

Fiber's Role

Under normal circumstances, all the carbohydrate sources such as starch and sugars are absorbed in the small intestine, along with all the protein and 95 percent of the fat. This leaves one large group of food-stuffs that has not been mentioned but is an important part of the diet: fiber.

Fiber is present in whole grains, fruits, vegetables, nuts, seeds, and dried beans (not meats or dairy products). Fiber is usually made up of complex carbohydrates or sugar residues that are *not* digestible by the enzymes from the pancreas and in the small intestine. Bacterial enzymes can break down fiber, however, and this is the next step in the digestion process.

Fiber is usually not released from the stomach until after a meal is completed and all digestible substances have been absorbed. The gut then changes its pattern of muscle contraction so that these food residues containing the fiber are emptied from the stomach and passed through the small intestine relatively quickly into the *large intestine*. Passing the fiber through separately keeps it from interfering with the normal absorption of nutrients. Still, fiber is absolutely crucial to normal large intestine function. Bacteria that live in the large intestine digest fiber using their own enzymes and nutrients from the breakdown. Gas can also be a by-product of this bacterial digestion of fiber. A diet lacking in fiber will often lead to further problems in large bowel activity.

The Body's Most Misunderstood Organ: The Colon

The large intestine or *colon* (see figure 3 on page 34) primarily absorbs the liquid that remains in the small intestine after the digestion and absorption of carbohydrates, fat, and protein. As the liquid is

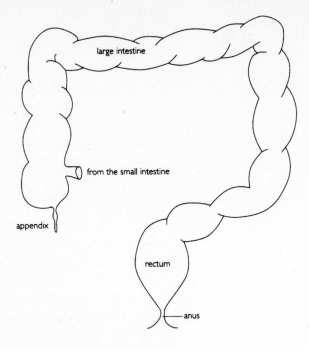

large intestine

from the small intestine

appendix

rectum

anus

Figure 3 The large intestine, or colon

reabsorbed, the colon forms the remaining materials into solid stool waste. Much of the stool is, in fact, made up of bacterial waste, because the colon normally houses large quantities of bacteria. Once the stool has been made into a more solid product, it is transported to the lower large intestine or *rectum*. Emptying of the stool occurs when you feel the stool in the rectum.

When irritable bowel causes the colon to be more sensitive, it does not work in a nice, coordinated manner. The contractions of the colon can be *irritable*, causing stool to move too quickly through the colon so that liquid isn't absorbed, which leads to diarrhea. The colon might also contract in a manner that prevents the stool from moving properly, causing constipation. Increased sensitivity in the colon can also make normal distension painful with irritable bowel, where other people would have little or no sensation with similar stretching of their colon. Although the gut appears to be normal, it just doesn't work the way a normal gut does.

Gut Timing

A common point of confusion is how long it normally takes foods to move through the gut. Food passes through the esophagus in a matter of seconds and is usually emptied to the stomach in under a minute. It may take as long as three or four hours after a meal before the stomach empties. Depending on the size and content of the meal, it could take even longer. Generally, high-fat meals take much longer to leave the stomach. After the stomach finishes emptying the food into the small intestine, the small intestine will take four to six hours to finish digesting the meal.

Recall that the fiber residues from a meal are broken down in the colon only after the small intestine is empty. When you consider the time it takes to digest meals, most people who eat three meals a day reach their "fasting state" (when there is no food left in the intestines to digest) during the night. It can take two to three days before material is finally packaged into stool and emptied from the rectum.

So why do people usually experience an urge to pass stool an hour or two after eating, or daily, or every two days? This is because nerve connections and reflexes trigger the large intestine to increase its activity, particularly the first thing in the morning so that the remaining food residues (stool) that have been stored for a day or two are moved into the rectum and evacuated. Colon function is most active first thing in the morning, after waking. This means that to achieve a regular bowel habit it is best to eat some food in the morning to help maximize stimulation of the colon. This is particularly true for people with constipation-predominant irritable bowel. Eating breakfast helps to get the colon active in the morning and reduces the likelihood of increased gas buildup and bloating throughout the day.

A "Thoughtful" Gut

The digestion process is incredibly complex. We have provided a simplified explanation in this chapter, but there are still many unanswered questions about its function. Nevertheless, the gut appears to be able to work without much input from the brain because it has its own "little brain." Complex nerve connections direct the gut through specific muscle contraction sequences depending on whether or not there is food in the intestines. Some evidence suggests that with irritable bowel the little brain has trouble coordinating the functions of the gut. Not surprisingly, this disruption could lead to symptoms typical of irritable bowel. In the next chapter, we will explain further how recent studies of irritable bowel have increased our understanding of how and why these troublesome symptoms occur in people who have irritable bowel.

4

What Causes Irritable Bowel?

A great deal of research has been devoted to discovering the causes of irritable bowel. We have learned a lot, but important questions still remain unanswered.

For many years, it was thought that irritable bowel was caused by abnormal *motility*, a term describing the coordinated contractions of the gut that move digested food and gas through the intestines as part of the digestion process. The bowel is like a big muscle that moves food and waste using a special type of muscular contractions called *peristaltic movements*. These contractions can be compared to the action necessary to retrieve a drawstring that has slipped into the waistband of your sweatpants. People with irritable bowel do sometimes have peristaltic movements that are poorly coordinated. However, research shows that this abnormal coordination does not always occur with irritable bowel symptoms. Another problem is that some people without irritable bowel also have erratic muscle contraction of the bowel, particularly in the large intestine. Therefore, differences in motility cannot completely explain the causes of irritable bowel. As a result, investigators began to look at other possible theories.

Is Irritable Bowel Inherited?

Our patients ask us this question all the time. Even though irritable bowel is very common, there haven't been many researchers who have studied whether or not irritable bowel is inherited. However, the few studies available do suggest that if you have irritable bowel, it is probable that your other family members have similar symptoms. This makes sense because we would expect that the reactivity of the bowel to food and other stimulation, such as stress, could be inherited from your parents. If other close family members have irritable bowel, it is possible but not certain that you will also develop these symptoms.

Some people with irritable bowel begin to have abdominal pain as children. Abdominal pain in children that is not associated with disease is common. Many children complain of abdominal pain if they are upset, if they don't want to go to school, and sometimes if they have other more serious complaints that are not related to the abdomen. In any case, if you have pain episodes when you are a child and no cause is found, there is about a 50 percent chance that you will develop irritable bowel when you reach adulthood. Again, this suggests that some people are predisposed to have irritable bowel.

Gut Hypersensitivity in Irritable Bowel

Recent studies suggest that irritable bowel occurs in individuals who have extremely sensitive intestines. Some sufferers also have a more sensitive stomach and esophagus (see chapter 3). In research studies, people with irritable bowel experienced much more pain when their bowel was stretched with a balloon. They also felt that their pain extended over a larger area of the abdomen compared to others whose bowels were distended. In other words, those with irritable bowel felt that their abdominal pain was more intense and widespread than those without irritable bowel. Studies of people with irritable bowel have shown that they tend to have a higher pain tolerance to other sources of pain such as electrical stimulation of the skin. People with irritable bowel don't just have a lower pain tolerance, their ability to withstand pain is actually increased—it is just their bowel pain that is more intense. Research also shows that people with irritable bowel experience muscle contractions in the intestines as painful or unpleasant, while these same contraction patterns go unnoticed by people without irritable bowel. Some of these contractions that are perceived as painful actually occur in the small intestine, rather than in the large intestine. Previously, the assumption was that most irritable bowel symptoms originated in the large intestine, so this new research emphasizes that the entire gut is sensitive with irritable bowel. This discovery has revolutionized our understanding of irritable bowel's underlying causes.

It appears that individuals with irritable bowel actually have increased perception of normal day-to-day activity in the gut such as food digestion and the movement of food waste through the intestines. Most people don't usually notice or react to gut activity, which suggests that irritable bowel is probably at the high end of a spectrum of intestinal awareness. Normal gut stimulation with irritable bowel can produce abnormal overreactions—the cardinal symptoms of irritable bowel (pain, altered bowel habits, mucus production, bloating, and sensations of incomplete rectal emptying).

Studies also show that loss of sleep will increase the intensity of irritable bowel symptoms. Because the brain controls sleeping and waking, these findings imply a link between the brain and the gut. Stressful events can also generate symptoms. Other studies also support the brain-gut connection, showing that when people with irritable bowel are placed in stressful situations, they experience definite abnormal contractions in the gut. More research is necessary, but it appears that the heightened sensitivity of the gut stems from underlying problems in the gut's nervous system or from altered nerve connections between the brain and the gut.

The Brain-Gut Connection and Its Role in Irritable Bowel

Research shows that when the gut is stimulated, there is more activity in the *emotional* and *alerting* areas of the brain in those who have irritable bowel compared to others who don't have it. These areas of the brain trigger responses such as our emotions and our alertness to possible threats. This explains one way in which the fight-or-flight system can be activated with irritable bowel (see chapter 8). This research shows us one reason that people with irritable bowel have such severe symptoms whereas others feel little or nothing in the same situation. The brain isn't diseased; it appears that the wiring or the nerve signals being sent to the brain are triggering responses that are stronger and overreact to what the nerve stimulation is actually from. Further research is needed to clarify whether this is primarily a problem with the nerves going from the gut to the brain, with the brain itself, or with the brain increasing the nerve signals sent to the brain by influencing the gut nerves directly. It will likely turn out to be a combination of these and other factors, with some people having more problems in one area than in others, yet all presenting with irritable bowel.

Studies of nerve function find that there may also be differences within the brain in people with irritable bowel and in the way they experience bowel symptoms. We know from several studies that the degree of distress that people experience will influence whether they seek medical advice for their irritable bowel symptoms. It may be that these individuals will magnify the intensity of the bowel symptoms experienced by the brain, due to the distress they are having. The ability of hypnosis to help some people with irritable bowel suggests that the brain may be one mechanism causing irritable bowel symptoms to be more severe. Hypnosis helps to lessen our response to outside influences, therefore modulating the overreaction in the brain response that triggers irritable bowel.

The Infection Connection

Beyond an overly sensitive gut, we know that irritable bowel can result from an infection of the intestines. Irritable bowel strikes approximately 30 percent of people who experience an infection that causes severe diarrhea. Irritable bowel symptoms can persist for years after the infection has cleared, or they may gradually fade over several months as normal bowel habit returns. Women appear to be more likely to develop irritable bowel after a severe intestinal infection; this could be one of the reasons women have irritable bowel more often than men.

Research into postinfectious irritable bowel finds that the nerves in the gut are sensitized by an infection and develop a "memory" of the disordered bowel function that is present when the infection has cleared. Studying the microscopic appearance of the bowel after the infection has cleared in people with postinfection irritable bowel shows some subtle changes in the nerves in the gut and an increased number of inflammatory cells around these nerves. There are also slight increases in other inflammatory cells in the bowel lining. These changes are so slight that they do not show up on the usual tests that look for such diseases as colitis or cancer. However, these slight changes do seem to be enough to explain the resulting bowel dysfunction after the infection has been cleared from the body.

Recent research has explored the use of probiotics in treating irritable bowel. Probiotics are good bacteria that live in the bowel and help maintain a healthy bowel lining, particularly the large bowel where most of the bacteria in the gut live (see chapter 3). At this time the research is incomplete, but a few studies have shown that some probiotic bacteria may provide benefit by reducing some bowel symptoms, especially bloating. Other studies have shown these benefits with only some probiotic bacteria and not others. It is too early to recommend taking probiotics until we know more about their effect in irritable bowel. They are not known to do harm, however, and these good bacteria may play a role in helping the intestine to recover after a serious intestinal infection.

So even after the infection is gone, symptoms similar to those caused by an infection persist (diarrhea, pain and cramping, mucus, and a feeling of incomplete rectal emptying). Again, symptoms caused by an infection can, in the short term, mimic those of irritable bowel. This is why your doctor cannot make a diagnosis of irritable bowel until the symptoms have been present for more than three months.

What about Food Allergy?

Many patients ask this question. *Food allergy* is very different from irritable bowel symptoms. If you have a food allergy, you will often develop a skin rash or feel shortness of breath and wheezing when you eat a food you are allergic to. This reaction can be life threatening: even a microscopic amount of the food can cause a severe reaction. Food allergy is often related to eggs, peanuts, and shellfish, but it can occur with other foods as well. If you have a food allergy, you should speak to your doctor about how to protect yourself, because you can accidentally eat something contaminated with the food you react to.

Irritable bowel does *not* cause this type of severe reaction when you eat an offending food. Some foods can certainly trigger irritable bowel, but these foods often do it in particular ways. Usually, the food contains some fiber that isn't digested in the small intestine (see chapter 3), and then bacteria metabolize the fiber and generate gas and other products of digestion that cause diarrhea, abdominal cramps, and gas and bloating symptoms. Some foods like flour (even white flour that has little fiber) can have small amounts of starch and/or protein that are not digested completely in the small intestine. These food residues are then broken down by the colonic bacteria, and abdominal cramping and gas result. Some people have the same reaction after they have consumed dairy products that have lactose (milk sugar) in them. These foods are not triggering an allergic reaction—they are just not completely digested, so the sensitivity in the colon from this extra bacterial digestion is provoking the symptoms. The symptoms are not an indication of any damage being done to the gut, though most people agree that the symptoms can be very unpleasant. If you think certain foods trigger your symptoms, be sure to read chapters 5, 6, and 7.

Using Science to Your Benefit

Though researchers do not yet know all the causes of irritable bowel, their work has led to better strategies for managing symptoms. For instance, understanding that your gut is more sensitive than normal may be useful as you monitor important aspects of your life. New medications have been (and are being) developed to help relieve some specific symptoms. Your doctor is a good resource to help manage your symptoms when they become particularly troublesome.

Think of your irritable bowel as an early warning system. When you experience your irritable bowel symptoms, take a moment to step back from what you are doing and evaluate what you have eaten or whether there are stressors that are affecting you. Your gut will let you know when your diet is less than ideal (for example, when you are consuming lots of high-fat foods or caffeine), and may help you identify when you are under stress so that you can respond in a positive and healthy manner. As you will read later on, knowing when you are under stress and what those stressors are will enable you to be proactive in controlling your irritable bowel.

Only about half of Americans with irritable bowel are diagnosed. People with less intense symptoms, particularly abdominal pain, are less likely to see a doctor. It may be that some of those with milder symptoms simply learn that certain foods or stressful situations trigger their symptoms, so they don't interpret them as being serious. By learning your own triggers, you, too, may be able to better control your symptoms and feel better with your irritable bowel. The following chapters will help you do just that.

5

Want Relief?
Start with Healthy Eating

Healthy eating is the first step in managing irritable bowel. This does not mean that you will be expected to become "virtuous" with your food choices (which is what many people think dietitians demand when they recommend a healthy diet). Instead, the advice in this chapter and the next is based on science and a good mix of professional and personal experience.

You see, dietitians tend to be drawn to their profession for the very reason that they like food. Most dietitians eat healthily, and their food choices include the occasional slice of pizza or a piece of cheesecake. There is a saying in the dietetic community: "All foods can fit," and they do. There are nutrient-dense foods (foods with plenty of nutrition and few calories) that we can eat lots of, and other foods that provide few nutrients and plenty of calories; we just eat these less frequently. We want to make this point at the beginning so you understand that our nutrition recommendations reflect optimal strategies for managing irritable bowel tempered with the appreciation that food is an important, if not focal, part of life. We recognize that eating is an important part of a healthy lifestyle for social reasons as much as for nutritional reasons.

Let's begin with a word of caution: no magic food or diet will cure your irritable bowel. You will hear claims that if you follow a special diet (often restrictive) or consume a specific product (often expensive), your irritable bowel will be cured. As you have read already in the earlier chapters of this book, irritable bowel is not actually a disease. Your bowel is normal, but easily irritated. Irritable bowel is never really cured, however. The symptoms are treated or managed through a variety of nutritional, psychological, and medical strategies as presented in this book.

When you have irritable bowel, there is a strong relationship between what you eat and how you feel. Instead of "you are what you eat," it should be "you *feel* what you eat." You probably know this already because you have had symptoms after eating certain foods. And you may have eliminated these foods from your diet only to have your symptoms persist. Unfortunately, there is more to managing symptoms of irritable bowel than removing foods from your diet. Read on, and we will take the mystery out of the malady.

In the next three chapters on nutrition, we will teach you how to manage your irritable bowel symptoms through healthy eating. There are three distinct steps to pursue. First, you will need to adopt healthy eating strategies to ensure that your food intake is healthy overall. Then, as you will learn in the next chapter, you will need to adjust your eating habits based on the eating-related causes of irritable bowel symptoms. These two steps are important, because you need adequate nutrition to feel well, function normally, and cope with stress. Also, you need to know your eating habits, which may be triggering symptoms, to manage irritable bowel effectively. Finally, in chapter 7 you will learn how to control your irritable bowel symptoms with specific diets. Following this three-step process is critical to managing your symptoms. If you skip the first or the second step, you will be disappointed, because the efforts you make may be less effective.

One final word before proceeding: there is a lot of material in this chapter and the next. You may want to read each chapter through once from beginning to end, then go back and work through each chapter again, this time more slowly.

Healthy Eating: You Feel What You Eat

To start off, we want to make the point that a healthy diet is a way of life or a lifestyle, not something you do one day (or week) and not the next. This is important to understand. As you will see, managing your irritable bowel symptoms will require you to make and stick with changes if you want to feel better. For many people, the word *diet* brings up images of a short-term food restriction plan to lose weight. We use the term *diet* to refer to any type of long-term eating plan that is designed to make you healthy or help you manage your irritable bowel symptoms. The diet changes we suggest may be challenging, but we are confident that you will find the rewards worth the effort. You will be in control of your symptoms!

Our discussion on healthy eating centers on MyPyramid (it replaces the Food Guide Pyramid), which is designed to help people, ages two years and older, choose a healthy diet and reduce their risk of chronic diseases. The Dietary Guidelines for Americans and the MyPyramid Food Guidance System, updated in 2005, are based on the preponderance of scientific evidence for lowering risk of chronic disease and promoting health.

The main health messages in MyPyramid are designed to improve the quality of the American diet. Specifically, people are advised to eat more fruits, vegetables, and whole grains; lower their intake of saturated fats, trans fats, and cholesterol; and balance calorie intake with output through regular physical activity to prevent weight gain and/or promote a healthy weight.

MyPyramid has Web-based interactive education materials for consumers. Visit www.MyPyramid.gov to learn about healthy food and activity choices personalized to fit your unique needs.

MyPyramid

MyPyramid provides direction on how to choose a healthy diet. It emphasizes choosing foods from five major food groups illustrated by the colorful sections in the pyramid: grains, vegetables, fruits, milk, and meats and beans.

All types of foods are represented in the pyramid, even those that should be eaten in limited quantities such as oils. Each food group provides specific nutrients, but not all the nutrients you need. For your health, you need to choose a variety of foods from all the food groups.

The Dietary Guidelines for Americans, MyPyramid, and the Nutrition Facts Panel on packaged foods use a 2,000-calorie diet as a reference for energy (calorie) and nutrient intake. Energy requirements vary with activity level, age, and gender. You may require more than 2,000 calories daily if you are young and/or active, significantly less if you are inactive and/or older (visit www.MyPyramid.gov to learn about your energy and nutrition requirements).

When we talk about healthy eating, we aren't referring to a single meal or one day. We are talking about your food intake over several days. Some days you may eat more vegetables than others, or more or less fat than others. If you are eating healthy, your intake should balance out over several days.

MyPyramid Concepts

The recommendations in the MyPyramid Food Guidance System fall under four general themes: variety, proportionality, moderation, and activity. These themes are discussed in the following sections in order to help you eat healthfully.

Variety

Selecting a variety of foods within and among the different food groups will ensure that you eat a variety of nutrients. This is very important to a healthy diet.

Variety is achieved by selecting foods from different food groups at each meal. Meals with variety contain three or more food groups. For example, a breakfast of cereal, low-fat milk, and juice represents three food groups. Lunch consisting of a sandwich filled with a lean meat, a glass of milk or yogurt, and a piece of fruit covers four food groups. A supper of lean meat; vegetables; whole wheat bread, pasta, or rice; a glass of milk; and a piece of fruit covers five food groups.

Proportionality

This term refers to eating more of some foods and less of others. Choose nutrient-dense foods—foods that provide lots of nutrients while at the

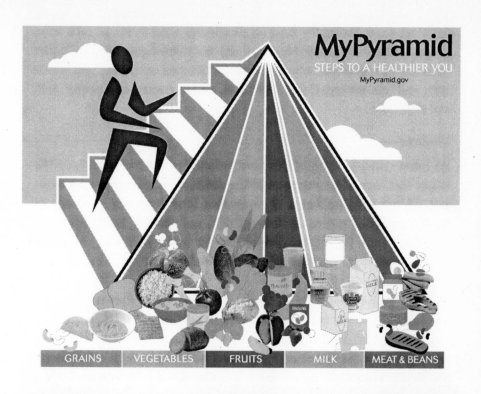

MyPyramid
STEPS TO A HEALTHIER YOU
MyPyramid.gov

| GRAINS | VEGETABLES | FRUITS | MILK | MEAT & BEANS |

GRAINS	VEGETABLES	FRUITS	MILK	MEAT & BEANS
Make half your grains whole	Vary your veggies	Focus on fruits	Get your calcium-rich foods	Go lean with protein
Eat at least 3 oz. of whole-grain cereals, breads, crackers, rice, or pasta every day 1 oz. is about 1 slice of bread, about 1 cup of breakfast cereal, or ½ cup of cooked rice, cereal, or pasta	Eat more dark-green veggies like broccoli, spinach, and other dark leafy greens Eat more orange vegetables like carrots and sweetpotatoes Eat more dry beans and peas like pinto beans, kidney beans, and lentils	Eat a variety of fruit Choose fresh, frozen, canned, or dried fruit Go easy on fruit juices	Go low-fat or fat-free when you choose milk, yogurt, and other milk products If you don't or can't consume milk, choose lactose-free products or other calcium sources such as fortified foods and beverages	Choose low-fat or lean meats and poultry Bake it, broil it, or grill it Vary your protein routine — choose more fish, beans, peas, nuts, and seeds

For a 2,000-calorie diet, you need the amounts below from each food group. To find the amounts that are right for you, go to MyPyramid.gov.

| Eat 6 oz. every day | Eat 2½ cups every day | Eat 2 cups every day | Get 3 cups every day; for kids aged 2 to 8, it's 2 | Eat 5½ oz. every day |

Find your balance between food and physical activity
- Be sure to stay within your daily calorie needs.
- Be physically active for at least 30 minutes most days of the week.
- About 60 minutes a day of physical activity may be needed to prevent weight gain.
- For sustaining weight loss, at least 60 to 90 minutes a day of physical activity may be required.
- Children and teenagers should be physically active for 60 minutes every day, or most days.

Know the limits on fats, sugars, and salt (sodium)
- Make most of your fat sources from fish, nuts, and vegetable oils.
- Limit solid fats like butter, margarine, shortening, and lard, as well as foods that contain these.
- Check the Nutrition Facts label to keep saturated fats, trans fats, and sodium low.
- Choose food and beverages low in added sugars. Added sugars contribute calories with few, if any, nutrients.

MyPyramid.gov
STEPS TO A HEALTHIER YOU

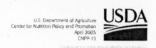

U.S. Department of Agriculture
Center for Nutrition Policy and Promotion
April 2005
CNPP-15

USDA

same time not too many calories. Recommended foods in each food group noted in this chapter represent nutrient-dense foods. Choose more fruits, vegetables, whole grains, and fat-free or low-fat milk products, and less saturated fats, trans fats, added sugars, cholesterol, salt, and alcohol.

Moderation

We know that you've heard this term before. Some substances should be in our diet in moderate amounts: fats, cholesterol, salt, sugars, caffeine, and alcohol. Choose forms of foods that limit intake of saturated or trans fats, added sugars, cholesterol, salt, and alcohol. For example, to moderate your fat intake, choose low-fat foods such as a baked or mashed potato rather than fried, or a whole wheat bagel instead of a croissant.

Many people think that if they eat a healthy diet they will become overweight. The key is to pay attention to portion sizes. Often, we eat a portion size that is more than a serving and think that it counts for one serving. Check the Nutrition Facts Panel or MyPyramid for the recommended portion size and compare it to the size of your portion.

Sometimes serving sizes are excessive. For example, according to MyPyramid, a restaurant-style plate of spaghetti and meatballs typically has four to six servings from the grains food group. Would you have thought of that meal providing so many servings of pasta? There is a portion distortion phenomenon in North America today, in which Americans don't have a sense of a reasonable portion size. We can safely reduce our portions and not sacrifice our nutritional health. In fact, our nutritional health improves as we are better able to achieve or maintain a healthy body weight. MyPyramid and the Nutrition Facts Panel will help you to gain a sense of a reasonable portion size.

Activity

Be physically active every day. Find balance between food and physical activity. If you feel that you cannot eat enough to get the nutrition you require, you need to be more physically active. Like nutrition, physical activity is key to your health and imperative to a healthy body weight. It is also a great way to reduce stress (chapter 9 includes more tips on stress management).

MyPyramid Particulars

MyPyramid divides foods into five groups based on their nutrient content. This section outlines the types of foods and amount recommended within each food group in order to have a healthy diet. Refer to MyPyramid on page 49. The key to the MyPyramid system is to find a balance between food intake and physical activity. Thirty to ninety minutes of daily physical activity is recommended, depending on whether you want to lose or maintain your weight. This level of physical activity represents a significant lifestyle change for many. Physical inactivity is a major reason why more than two-thirds of North Americans are overweight or obese. Consult www.MyPyramid.gov for advice on physical activity.

Grains Group

Any food made from wheat, rice, oats, cornmeal, barley, or another cereal grain is a grain product. Bread, pasta, oatmeal, breakfast cereals, and grits are examples of grain products. The grains group makes up the largest portion of the pyramid. Your body requires that most of your food choices come from these foods each day. This food group has plenty of complex carbohydrates (your body likes these starchy foods for fuel, particularly if they are low in fat), fiber, and B vitamins.

The grains group is particularly important to people with irritable bowel for two reasons. First, cereals and grains are a good source of fiber. Choosing whole grain products such as whole wheat bread, crackers, and bagels; cereals made from whole wheat or wheat bran; and muffins made with wheat bran will increase your fiber intake significantly. (Chapter 7 contains a lengthy discussion on a high-fiber diet, because it is the major diet adjustment for people with constipation-prone irritable bowel.) The second important point is that people with irritable bowel tend to tolerate breads, cereals, rice, and pasta well. In other words, these foods generally cause no or minimal irritable bowel symptoms. However, we caution you about what you put on starchy foods. For example, you may not tolerate a spicy tomato sauce with pasta or a spicy curry dish over rice.

Many people believe that foods in the grains group are fattening. For the most part this is just not true. It is what we put on these foods or how we prepare them that increases the calorie content. Opt to use small amounts of margarine or butter on bread, decrease the cream sauce you put on pasta, and know that frying rice adds fat to the grain. Remember: there is just as much fat in margarine as in butter, and both of these foods can provoke symptoms of irritable bowel if eaten in large quantities.

Some people try to increase their fiber intake by selecting bran muffins from a bakery or doughnut shop. These baked goods are often high in fat and sugar and hence calories. If you are concerned about weight gain, we caution you about buying these foods, as it may result in an excessive calorie intake and increased weight. We advise you to bake muffins (see our high-fiber, low-fat recipes in the appendix), buy a low-fat mix, or select low-fat varieties at the bakery. Also, you can always choose other low-fat, low-calorie, fiber-containing foods.

The guidelines recommend that half of your grain choices contain whole grain (at least three whole grain choices). We advise you to make all your choices whole grain if you require a high-fiber diet (see chapter 7 to determine if you need a high-fiber diet). The following list breaks down healthy versus not-so-healthy grain choices:

Healthy Choices	Not-So-Healthy Choices
Whole wheat bread	Croissant
Whole wheat bagel	Cheese bread
Whole wheat pita bread	Cheese biscuit
Low-fat whole wheat crackers	Garlic bread
Steamed brown rice	Fried plain rice
Whole wheat pasta or noodles	White pasta or noodles
Low-fat muffins	Sweets

How much should I eat from the grains group daily? Six to eleven 1-ounce equivalents. People on a 2,000-calorie diet are in the lower range of servings. One slice of bread, 1 cup of ready-to-eat cereal, or ½ cup of cooked rice, cooked pasta, or cooked cereal are considered as 1-ounce equivalents from the grains group.

Vegetables Group

The vegetables group provides a lot of nutrition, primarily vitamins A and C and folate, along with minerals such as iron and magnesium. Vegetables are low in fat, as long as they are prepared and eaten without added fat. Vegetables are also a good source of fiber. Choosing a variety of vegetables provides you with a variety of nutrients. The Dietary Guidelines for Americans recommend that you eat more dark green vegetables such as broccoli, spinach, and other leafy greens and choose more orange vegetables such as carrots and sweet potatoes. Some vegetables are more gas forming than others. (If you experience gas and bloating, refer to the low-gassy foods diet in chapter 7 to learn which vegetables you tolerate best.)

Legumes such as navy beans, pinto or kidney beans, and chickpeas are in two food groups because they are a good source of the nutrients found in both the vegetables group (fiber, vitamins, and minerals) and the meat group (protein). If you count them as a vegetable serving, they do not count as a protein choice at the same time.

The vegetables group is divided into five parts based on their nutrient content.

1. **Dark green vegetables**
   Bok choy
   Dark green leafy lettuce
   Mesclun greens
   Romaine lettuce
   Spinach
   Turnip greens

2. **Orange vegetables**
   Acorn squash
   Butternut squash
   Carrots
   Pumpkin
   Sweet potatoes

3. **Legumes**
   Black beans
   Black-eyed peas
   Garbanzo beans (chickpeas)
   Kidney beans
   Lentils
   Split peas

4. **Other vegetables**
   Artichokes
   Asparagus
   Beets
   Cabbage
   Cauliflower
   Celery
   Cucumbers
   Green beans
   Green and red peppers
   Iceberg lettuce
   Mushrooms
   Onions
   Parsnips
   Tomatoes
   Vegetable juice

5. **Starchy vegetables**
   Corn
   Green peas
   Potatoes

For people who have gas and bloating, we often recommend that particular vegetables be avoided or limited because of their gas-producing potential.

How much should I eat from the vegetables group daily? Two and a half cups per day for a person on a 2,000-calorie diet. One cup of raw or cooked vegetables or vegetable juice, or 2 cups of raw leafy greens are considered as 1 cup from the vegetables group.

Fruits Group

Fruits and fruit juices have varied amounts of vitamins and minerals—in particular, vitamins A and C, potassium, and fiber. As with the vegetables group, choosing a variety of fruits is important to get the nutrition you need. Certain fruits are particularly gas forming and may need to be limited or avoided to control gas and bloating symptoms.

How much should I eat from the fruits group daily? Two cups per day for a 2,000-calorie diet. One cup of fruit or 100 percent fruit juice; a small apple, peach, pear, or banana; or ½ cup of dried fruits are considered as 1 cup from the fruits group.

Milk Group

Milk products provide calcium, protein, riboflavin, potassium, phosphorus, and vitamins A and D. In short, this food group is loaded with nutrition. Without milk products in your diet, it would be difficult to get enough calcium for your bone health. For more information on milk products and irritable bowel and calcium requirements and supplements, see "Lactose: The Suspected Sugar" in chapter 7.

Consuming milk, cheese, or yogurt is often an issue for people with digestive problems because they are frequently told to avoid milk products as a means to reduce their gastrointestinal symptoms. This can lead to unnecessarily avoiding milk products. It's true that lactose or natural milk sugar may not be completely digested in some individuals and cause gas, bloating, and diarrhea. Lactose intolerance is not an element of irritable bowel, but in some people the symptoms are similar. Milk, cheese, and yogurt contain fat. You can reduce the fat you get from this food group, however, by choosing lower-fat items such as fat-free or 1 percent milk, fat-reduced cheese, and yogurt made with fat-reduced milk.

Some dairy products don't belong in this food group and should be limited because they are high in fat and provide few vitamins and minerals and little protein. Butter, cream, and cream cheese have little or no calcium and are not part of this group. They should be used sparingly.

How much should I eat from the milk group daily? Three cups per day. One cup of milk or yogurt, 1½ ounces of natural cheese, or 2 ounces of processed cheese are each considered as 1 cup from the milk group. Choose low-fat or fat-free milk, yogurt, and other milk products.

Meat and Beans Group

Meat, poultry, fish, and eggs provide protein, B vitamins, iron, and zinc. Dried beans, peas, and nuts provide similar nutrients and are good sources of complex carbohydrates and fiber (and can also be counted in the vegetables group).

Dried beans, peas, and nuts can worsen the irritable bowel symptoms of abdominal gas and bloating; therefore, we recommend that people with these symptoms limit or avoid these foods. Unfortunately, avoiding dried beans, peas, and nuts may be problematic for vegetarians and particularly vegans (who don't eat meat, fish, poultry, eggs, and cheese). If you are a vegetarian and you want to control gas and bloating symptoms, we advise you to see a dietitian or nutrition professional, who can give you advice on how to get proper nutrition.

Meat can contain a significant amount of fat. You can keep the fat content of your diet lower by choosing leaner cuts of meat. Examples of lean cuts of meat include round, loin, and sirloin beef; center loin; tenderloin pork; ham; and chicken or turkey without the skin.

How much should I eat from the meat and beans group daily? Five-and-a-half-ounce equivalents per day for a 2,000-calorie diet. One ounce of lean meat, poultry, or fish, 1 egg, 1 tablespoon of peanut butter, ¼ cup cooked dry beans or ½ ounce of nuts or seeds are *each* considered a 1-ounce equivalent from the meat and beans group.

Oils Group

The food group from which we need the smallest amount is the oils group. Oils are fats that are liquid at room temperature, such as the vegetable oils used in cooking. Common oils are canola, corn, olive, safflower, and soybean. Foods that are mainly oils include mayonnaise, certain salad dressings, and soft tub or squeeze margarine with no trans fat. Oils from vegetables do not contain cholesterol. However, a few plant oils, including coconut oil and palm kernel oil, are high in saturated fat, and for this reason they are considered solid fats and should be used very sparingly.

Solid fats are solid at room temperature and include butter, shortening, beef fat, chicken fat, pork fat, and solid margarine. You should limit the solid fats in your diet as well as foods that contain these fats.

Trans fats are also solid at room temperature. They are produced when liquid vegetable oils are hydrogenated (hydrogen is whipped into the oil, making it solid). Trans fats elevate the "bad" cholesterol that increases your risk of coronary heart disease and should be used very sparingly. Trans fats are commonly found in processed foods that contain partially hydrogenated vegetable oils such as vegetable shortening, some margarines (especially more solid margarines), crackers, candies, cookies, snack foods, fried foods, and baked goods. To minimize your intake of fat that increases your cholesterol level, check the Nutrition Facts Panel on packaged foods. Choose foods with lower amounts of saturated fat, trans fat, and cholesterol.

How much should I eat from the oils group daily? Most people consume enough oil in the foods they eat, such as salad dressings, cooking oil, fish, and nuts. A person's allowance for oils depends on their age, gender, and level of physical activity. MyPyramid suggests an allowance of 5 to 6 teaspoons per day for women, and 6 to 7 teaspoons per day for men.

Discretionary Calories

The MyPyramid system also includes a category called *discretionary calories*. These calories are extras that you can eat once you meet your nutrient requirements from the recommended choices under each food group. Types of foods in the discretionary category are solid fats, added sugars, alcohol, or more food from any group. Your discretionary calorie allowance depends on your energy needs, and most allowances are very small: between 100 and 300 calories per day, especially for people who are not physically active. Often, the discretionary calorie allowance is used up by food choices such as higher-fat meats, cheeses, milk, or bakery items.

Snack Attack Strategies

It's four in the afternoon, the time of day when you're most hungry. You're at the office, and you've got to have something to eat. What is going to satisfy your hunger and at the same time not increase your irritable bowel symptoms?

Contrary to what many people believe, snacking can be a part of a healthy diet. In fact, with irritable bowel your gut may tolerate smaller meals and in-between-meal snacks better than it does a few large meals. Just make sure you choose healthy snacks and guard against over-consuming calories or fat.

Some snacks we know to be healthy are not tolerated well by people with irritable bowel. For example, low-fat popcorn and raw vegetables should be avoided if you have problems with gas and bloating. These snacks are particularly troublesome when consumed on an empty stomach.

If you are concerned that snacking may lead to weight gain, there are plenty of other low-calorie snacks, even if you cannot eat raw vegetables. Look for low-fat starchy foods such as low-fat whole wheat crackers or baby crackers. Besides being low in calories and fat, they are well tolerated. Weight gain can also be avoided by keeping the size of your snack small; use the Nutrition Facts Panel to determine the size of one serving.

In general, starchy foods such as breads, crackers, and cereal are well tolerated. The ideal starchy snack would contain whole wheat or wheat bran. Other foods such as milk, low-fat cheese or yogurt, fruit or fruit juice, or smooth peanut butter also tend to be well tolerated and may be combined with a whole wheat starchy item.

Healthy Snacks If You Have Irritable Bowel

- Low-fat wheat bran muffin (small). Pass on the margarine or butter.
- Cereal and low-fat milk (the best cereal choice is made with whole wheat). This is an excellent snack because it is low in fat (except granola-type cereals) and includes calcium-rich milk.
- Low-fat whole wheat crackers, plain or with low-fat cheese or peanut butter. Eating only a few low-fat crackers can help you through a hungry period such as during meal preparation or the drive home after work.

- Low-fat yogurt. This is a good snack because it is calcium rich and usually very well tolerated. Try various brands and flavors to decide which tastes the best. You may want to try a yogurt with probiotic (live bacterial culture) bacteria, which may decrease bloating symptoms (see chapter 4).
- Digestive, fruit-filled, or baby cookies. These snacks do not contain significant fiber, but they are well tolerated.
- Fresh fruit that you know you can tolerate. Fruits generally tolerated are peeled apples, ripe pears, peaches, and nectarines (when the skin and fruit is soft).
- Canned fruit. This is a well-tolerated snack. Choose fruit packed in its own juice without added sugar.
- Pretzels and low-fat potato snacks or rice cakes.
- Whole wheat toast. Use a very small amount of margarine or butter or try jam, low-fat cheese, or peanut butter. Make cinnamon toast by spreading on a small amount of margarine or butter and sprinkling with cinnamon sugar.
- Frozen yogurt. This is a good replacement for ice cream. Try the many different flavors and brands.
- Baked potato. This is a great choice for a warm snack. Try it plain or with a very small amount of margarine, butter, or sour cream. Another option is to add a small amount of grated cheddar or Parmesan cheese.
- Rice. Rice is well tolerated by people with irritable bowel. Make a snack out of leftover whole grain rice with a small amount of margarine or butter or leftover rice casserole.
- Pudding. This calcium-rich choice is healthy as long as it is made with low-fat milk and with little added sugar. Rice and bread pudding are also possible choices.

Eating Out: Pleasure or Pain?

Eating out is often a dilemma for people with irritable bowel. Should you eat whatever you please and pay the consequences later? Or should you look over the menu carefully and pick items that will likely provoke the fewest, if any, irritable bowel symptoms? You may choose to "go for it" on some occasions and be cautious on others. Our advice is that if you eat out frequently (more than twice a week), you should choose menu items based on what you know you tolerate and like.

If you eat out infrequently, you might consider any discomfort you experience from eating foods that provoke irritable bowel symptoms well worth it. We don't disagree with this choice; we appreciate how you feel. You just need to prepare yourself for the symptoms. You won't damage your bowels, but you will make your symptoms worse and your life miserable. Managing symptoms is what this book is all about; therefore, we cannot recommend that you eat any offending food on a frequent (daily or every other day) basis. But once in a while might be worth it. This is especially true when you take into consideration how much of our eating is social.

Most people choose a restaurant based on what they feel like eating and price. We suggest that you add another consideration: whether the menu includes items that you can tolerate with minimal or no symptoms. It makes plenty of sense to choose a restaurant that offers menu items that will not trigger irritable bowel symptoms.

Tips for Pleasurable Eating Out

- Don't be timid about asking your server how a food is prepared or that a menu item be prepared in a lean way if it is usually fried or served in a cream sauce. Your server wants you to be pleased with your meal. You may even inspire a change to more lean preparation techniques in the restaurant.
- Choose tomato sauce rather than cream sauce. Tomato sauce usually has little added fat. If you have heartburn, ask that a small amount of cream sauce be added, or request it on the side.
- Look for menu items that are prepared in low-fat ways—baked, broiled, charbroiled, barbecued, stir-fried, poached, roasted, grilled, steamed, and braised. Healthy, hot meals that are generally well-tolerated include:

  Charbroiled chicken or steak

  Grilled, broiled, or poached fish

  Baked or mashed potatoes or steamed rice

  Cooked vegetables

- Check the menu for sandwiches. Depending on the toppings, sandwiches are usually well tolerated if you have irritable bowel. Request whole wheat bread or a whole wheat bagel to increase your fiber intake. If you have gas and bloating, skip sandwiches that are loaded with vegetables such as cucumbers, lettuce, or tomatoes. Opt for a leaf or two of lettuce if you want to avoid irritable bowel symptoms.
- Always request salad dressing on the side and use small amounts; however, you need to know that salad may increase gas and bloating symptoms.
- For dessert choose frozen yogurt, sorbet, angel food cake, fruit salad (avoid citrus if you have heartburn, and melons or unpeeled apples if you have gas and bloating).
- If you are eating out in a fast-food restaurant, check the menu for healthy choices. The fast-food industry has caught on that its customers want healthy options, so you should be able to purchase healthy food no matter which major fast-food chain you choose.

Weight-Loss Diets: Winning at the Game of Losing

Excess weight has become an epidemic in North America, with two-thirds of North Americans either overweight or obese. It is likely that people with irritable bowel are among the many who struggle to achieve and maintain a healthy body weight. If you would like to know how to select a weight-loss eating strategy that will help you to keep the weight you lose off, as well as remove potential triggers to your irritable bowel symptoms, read on.

Most of you who want to lose weight have tried many types of diets in the past, with limited success. You have lots of company. There is no shortage of choice when it comes to weight-loss diets. The weight-loss industry has kept pace with the rate of obesity with little or no effect on the problem. Many new diets promise weight loss, some suggesting you will never be hungry, others saying you can eat all you want. Sound too good to be true? It is. There just is no magic to weight loss and weight management, just a straightforward equation: if you eat more calories than you need or burn off, you will gain weight. If you eat fewer, you will lose weight. If you eat the amount of calories that you require, you will maintain weight.

So what do you try next: the "New" Atkins, the South Beach, the Zone, Dr. Phil's Ultimate Weight Solution, or the Glycemic Index Diet? Have you tried a number of these? Did the diets work a little bit, but then become too difficult to stick with, or did they result in limited weight loss? Why don't you evaluate what you know of these diets against criteria for an effective and healthy weight-loss program and answer the following questions. You may learn why the diets you have tried don't work.

There are three pillars to any good weight-loss program. A healthy weight-loss program will:

1. Provide adequate nutrition. The diet should include a variety of foods from all five food groups. Compare diet recommendations with the MyPyramid guidelines. If a food group is excluded, beware: the diet is compromising your health. MyPyramid is based on years of scientific research on our nutritional requirements. Your nutrition and health will be compromised if you eliminate an entire food group.

2. *Promote physical activity.* Exercise is key to weight loss, weight maintenance, and overall health. It is as important as a healthy diet, if not more so. Exercise allows you to eat more while in weight-loss and weight-maintenance phases. It has many other beneficial effects on our health—mental, physical, and spiritual. What a deal exercise is! A diet program that does not promote exercise is doing you a disservice.

3. *Provide education about behavior modification or lifestyle change.* In other words, a good weight-loss program supports you in learning strategies that help you to successfully lose *and* maintain weight loss. For example, does the program suggest ways for you to become aware of and avoid your triggers for eating excessively? Does the program offer ways that you can start new healthy eating habits to replace the old ones? Developing a lifestyle that includes healthy eating and physical activity to achieve and maintain a healthy body weight should be the goal of any credible weight-loss program.

The following are a few additional things to consider when selecting a weight-loss program:

- *Does the program recommend a weight loss of no more than 2 pounds per week?* A weight loss of 2 pounds or less per week is safe and reasonable. Quick weight loss or near starvation results in your body's metabolism slowing down to conserve energy, hence your body adapts and needs less energy to function. You may in fact end up heavier after the diet because you require less energy than you did before the severe calorie restriction.

- *Does the diet set realistic goal weights?* Some diets set unrealistically low goal weights based on a culturally prescribed desire for extreme thinness. Goal weights should be determined based on what is good for your health. The best method available to determine a healthy body weight is the body mass index (BMI). This index has been used in research for many years and is a better predictor of healthy body weights than the traditional height and weight ratios (at your height, you should weigh . . .). The calculation provides a healthy weight range for you and is easy to calculate:

$$BMI = 705 \times body\ weight\ /\ (height \times height)$$

For example, a person who is five feet, six inches (66 inches) tall and weighs 155 pounds would calculate BMI as:

$$BMI = 705 \times 155\ /\ (66 \times 66) = 25$$

You may use the following guidelines to interpret your BMI:

If your BMI is:	You are:
Less than 18.5	Underweight
18.5–24.9	Healthy weight
25–29.9	Overweight
30 and above	Obese

Another quick way to find out whether you have a healthy body weight is to measure your waist circumference. People carry weight on their body in two ways:

1. On their torso and around their middle (apple shaped)
2. On their hips, thighs, and bottoms (pear shaped)

People who are apple shaped, particularly if they are over-weight (their BMI equals 25 or greater), are at increased risk of developing heart disease, diabetes, high blood pressure, and high cholesterol.

To measure your waist circumference, wrap a tape measure around the narrowest part of your torso. Men should measure at their navel (belly button) and women should measure midway between the bottom of the ribs and the top of the hip bones. Be sure that the tape is snug. Relax, exhale and measure your waist.

Women who have a waist circumference greater than 35 inches are at increased risk for the chronic diseases mentioned earlier, and men who have a waist circumference greater than 40 inches are at increased risk of chronic disease. In Asians, these measurements are even smaller; women with a waist circumference greater than 32 inches and men with a waist circumference greater than 36 inches are at increased risk.

- *Does the program provide at least 1,200 calories for women and 1,500 calories for men?* If a diet provides fewer calories than this, then you will find it very difficult to get the nutrients you need and to stick with the plan, as lower calorie intakes represent severe restrictions in food intake.
- *Does the diet depend on special products, foods, or supplements?* If special foods or products are recommended, that should be a red flag for you. If the diet has enough calories (see the previous question), special products and supplements are not required. There is no substitute for nutritious, wholesome foods.
- *Does the program make any magical claims?* Magical claims are just that—magical. If it sounds too good to be true, it is. For some reason in our culture, eating healthy, wholesome foods and enjoying physical activity are not sexy and are totally unmarketable as a means to achieve and maintain a healthy body weight. Yet, this is precisely what is needed to achieve this goal.

An important consideration for people with irritable bowel is whether they will tolerate the foods recommended on a diet. Many weight-loss diets recommend lots of salads, raw vegetables, and snacking on popcorn. These types of foods worsen the symptoms of gas and bloating. Your best bet, if you have gas and bloating, is to follow the low gassy foods diet in chapter 7 as well as the weight-loss diet if you wish to feel better. The suggested snacks and eating-out food choices in this chapter tend to be well tolerated by people with gas and bloating.

Some weight-loss diets, particularly those that severely restrict carbohydrates, are very low in fiber. Fiber is recommended for irritable bowel sufferers with constipation or with alternating constipation and diarrhea. As noted earlier, eliminating a food group is a red flag for a weight-loss diet that is not healthy. If you feel that you must be on a weight-loss diet that is low in fiber, take a bulking agent such as Metamucil or Prodiem and drink plenty of water. Guidelines on how to introduce a high-fiber diet or a bulking agent into your diet are found in chapter 7.

6

Foods and Habits
That Irritate

Now that you understand how to adopt a healthy, balanced diet by using MyPyramid, you are ready to look at how your diet—the foods you choose to eat and how you choose to eat them—may be provoking or aggravating your symptoms. Later in the chapter, we provide strategies to remedy these diet-related causes.

Dietary aggravators of irritable bowel fit into three general categories:

1. *Eating patterns.* This refers to how you eat (when, where, how often, and how fast) and is closely related to your lifestyle, for example, whether you tend to eat breakfast or frequently eat at fast-food restaurants.

2. *Symptom-provoking foods.* This is what you eat. Many people report that even though they do not experience symptoms, they are unable to tolerate certain foods. Fatty, gassy, or spicy foods are often singled out, although there are a few hidden ingredients in other foods that can provoke irritable bowel symptoms (see pages 106 and 107).

Eating patterns relate to symptom-provoking foods in a complex way. It is not only how much you eat but whether you eat two or more symptom-provoking foods at once, or eat one or more at one meal and one or more at the next. All these factors will have a bearing on whether you experience irritable bowel symptoms.

3. *Insufficient fiber and water.* If you have constipation-predominant irritable bowel, all experts agree that a major aggravator of irritable bowel symptoms is insufficient fiber and water in the diet. We have seen this in our practice, too. By far the majority of people with constipation-prone irritable bowel and alternating bowel habit referred to us do not have enough fiber and water in their diets.

Taking a Closer Look at the Symptom Aggravators

Your lifestyle plays an important role in inciting your irritable bowel symptoms. It is important for you to identify whether eating patterns, symptom-provoking foods, and/or insufficient amounts of fiber and water are the cause of your symptoms. This is one of the first steps in gaining control over irritable bowel. The most important point to realize is that the symptom-producing patterns or habits can be changed and that you are in control of that change. Later in this chapter we will review some general guidelines regarding eating patterns that will help you keep your irritable bowel symptoms to a minimum.

Eating Patterns

Some symptoms of irritable bowel are related to a person's lifestyle. Many of us find that we are too busy to take good care of our nutritional needs. Furthermore, a busy lifestyle often means a stressful lifestyle. Irritable bowel symptoms are more pronounced when you are stressed (see chapter 8). Perhaps you can appreciate this from your own experience. When you feel stressed, you should pay particular attention to your eating habits to make sure your symptoms remain under control. There are several common problems regarding eating patterns that we see in people with irritable bowel.

Eating Food Fast

Eating too quickly or on the run can result in indigestion. Indigestion refers to feelings of discomfort in your stomach, bloating, reflux (stomach contents refluxing back up your esophagus), and heartburn. This can result from eating too quickly because your gastrointestinal tract does not have the ability to deal with the food in such a short time frame.

Eating Fast Food

A busy lifestyle, convenience, or just a liking for fast food may cause people with irritable bowel to consume meals of pizzas, burgers, fries, or fried chicken from fast-food outlets. These foods tend to be hard to digest for anyone and particularly people with irritable bowel. Because these foods are usually high in fat, this often leads to indigestion, abdominal pain, and even diarrhea. There may also be other ingredients in fast food such as preservatives that cause symptoms of irritable bowel. Whether the cause is high-fat content or another ingredient, generally, fast foods are difficult to digest.

Skipping Meals

Skipping meals or erratic eating habits (eating one meal per day or eating lots one day and little the next) provoke irritable bowel symptoms, particularly gas. Other symptoms caused by skipping meals include bloating, abdominal pain, and irregular bowel movements. Skipping meals may be related to a busy lifestyle. People might work through lunch, or parents busy with child care or elder care responsibilities might not take the time to eat. Many women skip meals or eat a lot one day and little the next as a weight-control strategy. Unfortunately, it doesn't work. It does, however, make irritable bowel symptoms all the worse. Studies show that the skipped meal or the low-calorie day is more than compensated for by consuming more food at other times. The pattern of not eating and then eating lots also triggers the body to store more energy as fat, thus defeating the weight-loss strategy.

Eating Junk Food

Junk food is high in calories and fat and provides very few nutrients. Examples of junk food are potato chips, nachos, cheese puffs, and chocolate bars. People with irritable bowel who treat themselves to a nighttime snack of potato chips, nachos, or some other type of high-fat food will likely find it hard to digest. High-fat snacks may result in indigestion, gas, diarrhea, and/or abdominal pain.

Overeating

The amount of food eaten at one time is a critical point to consider. North Americans tend to overeat. Eating is at the center of most celebrations. We like to eat out and are doing this on an ever-increasing basis. This is particularly problematic when the restaurant of choice offers large portions, contributing to our overeating and portion distortion, where we lose a sense of reasonable portion size. Some people have a tendency to overeat when they are stressed because they use eating as a means of comfort and nurturing. Independently, stress and overeating aggravate your symptoms of irritable bowel. Together, the effects are even greater. People with irritable bowel do not tolerate eating in excess very well. With overeating comes indigestion, bloating, abdominal pain, and nausea, particularly if the meal is high in fat.

Symptom-Provoking Foods

Many people with irritable bowel do not digest fatty, gassy, or spicy foods well. These symptom-provoking foods and other poorly tolerated foods are called *trigger foods*. (See chapter 7 to find out which foods are fatty, gassy, and spicy.) These trigger foods may result in a variety of symptoms such as gas, bloating, diarrhea, and abdominal pain. In addition, there are many not-so-obvious trigger foods: for instance, food or drink that is high in caffeine. Caffeine causes frequent bowel movements in people who are prone to diarrhea, induces pain (from increased bowel contractions or spasms), and is a major cause of heartburn.

We noted earlier that how much you eat of a trigger food—whether you eat one or more of these foods at once or several throughout the day—will have a bearing on the severity of your irritable bowel symptoms. Unfortunately, the effects of trigger foods are often unpredictable, making it all the more perplexing for someone trying to sort out the mysteries of their symptoms.

Many people come to us feeling very frustrated because they have not been able to pin down the problem foods. In fact, their frustration is so great that they have given up trying to figure out what they can and cannot eat. This is an example of how irritable bowel can cause stress. Identifying trigger foods is indeed challenging. Some people have learned to avoid certain foods, but if other trigger foods remain in their diet, their symptoms will continue. Others attempt a high-fiber diet not knowing that fiber needs to be introduced gradually, that certain fibers make you feel gassy and don't help your bowel habit all that much, or that fiber does not work when you are not drinking enough water. Needless to say, these people arrive in our clinic feeling pretty lousy and frustrated. When they start to follow our advice, however, their symptoms improve dramatically.

A common lament goes like this: "I was at a party the other night, and I was concerned whether I could eat what was being offered. I was relieved when I saw that there was lasagna, Caesar salad, and rolls. The last time I had lasagna I tolerated it fine, so I took some. I've had a problem with Caesar salad in the past, so I had only a very tiny amount. Not long after, I was never so sick! I left early and was kept awake with gas, bloating, and diarrhea."

It's frustrating, but you may be able to tolerate a certain food at one time and not at another. Caesar salad (fatty and gassy) and spaghetti or lasagna (potentially gassy, spicy, and fatty) are examples of foods that you may tolerate only occasionally. Even your mother's turkey dinner (potentially fatty and possibly including a spicy stuffing) may represent a meal that you would tolerate only occasionally.

Usually, if a situation is examined, a circumstance or two can be identified that contributed to the irritable bowel symptoms. For instance, for the person who attended the party, we would have asked whether she had any wine or other alcohol with her meal. Did she eat paté or some other fatty appetizer that she forgot about? Was she stressed or excited? What did she have for lunch? What did she eat the previous day? Quite often, when we examine the larger picture, we can understand why symptoms flared up. There are instances, however, when we cannot determine the cause of a person's symptoms. You will experience situations like this. Don't be dismayed, though; they occur fewer and fewer times when you learn what foods trigger your symptoms and the effective nutritional strategies to correct them.

In order for you to learn which foods are causing your symptoms, your diet and symptoms need to be examined in light of factors such as how much you ate of a potential trigger food and if you ate additional symptom-provoking foods with it, earlier in the day, or the day before. An important nonnutritional consideration is whether you are stressed. People with irritable bowel will always be more symptomatic when under stress. This is a general truth about the condition. Stress management is an important adjunct to nutritional management of irritable bowel symptoms for most people. Chapter 9 contains useful, practical guidelines on how to manage stress.

The amount of a potential trigger food a person can eat before experiencing symptoms depends on the particular food—and the person. Some foods, even if consumed in small amounts, provoke symptoms in most everyone with irritable bowel. Baked beans, pizza, and ice cream are common trigger foods. Some people with irritable bowel can tolerate small amounts of these and other trigger foods, but over a certain level of intake, symptoms occur. Coffee is another example of a trigger food that may not be tolerated at all, or just in small amounts, perhaps only one cup per day. It is clear, however, that people with irritable bowel will not tolerate excessive amounts of coffee—three or more mugs a day (6 to 8 ounces each)—without experiencing symptoms.

How often a trigger food is eaten has implications for irritable bowel symptoms. You might be able to tolerate certain foods occasionally if you don't eat too much at once. Fatty, gassy, or spicy foods fall into this category. For example, some people prone to gas can eat a small side salad with a meal and tolerate this fine if they eat it only once or twice a week. Also, some people can eat a fatty food such as a fast-food burger, if they don't eat it more than once every week or two (and don't eat fatty french fries with it). Some patients tell us that they can tolerate the occasional bowl of moderately spicy chili fine, but that they don't dare eat it two nights in a row (and they don't eat it with a gassy salad or a side of refried beans).

Not-So-Obvious Trigger Ingredients

We mentioned earlier that there are ingredients in foods that most people do not know can cause irritable bowel symptoms. The first is fructose, the natural sugar found in fruits and berries. Fructose has been shown to increase abdominal distress in people with irritable bowel.

The symptoms are primarily gas, bloating, and diarrhea, and they appear to be related to bacteria in the large intestine that digest natural sugar not completely absorbed in the small intestine. Apple juice, which is naturally high in fruit sugar, may be one of the causes of chronic diarrhea in children and adults. We see a fair number of people with diarrhea who consume six or more 8-ounce glasses of juice per day. When we ask them to decrease their intake to no more than one or two glasses daily, their diarrhea resolves.

The second substance that may worsen your irritable bowel symptoms is soft drinks, which contain large amounts of sugar. Large quantities of sugar are not well digested and result in diarrhea. We see people with diarrhea who have a 2-liter-per-day soft drink habit. The diarrhea is often further aggravated by the fact that the soft drink of choice tends to be a cola (dark) that contains caffeine. Again, when we advise these individuals to decrease their soft drink intake to no more than one or two 8-ounce glasses per day, their diarrhea subsides.

The third substance that can trigger irritable bowel symptoms is sorbitol. Sorbitol is found in a variety of fruits and plants and is used as a low-calorie sweetener because it is not well digested. But this same property might produce symptoms of indigestion such as gas, bloating, diarrhea, and abdominal pain. Common foods containing significant amounts of sorbitol include peaches, apple juice, pears, sugarless gum, dietetic jams, and dietetic chocolate.

Another dietary constituent that might cause irritable bowel symptoms is olestra, a calorie-free fat substitute made from vegetable oils and sugar. Look for olestra's brand name, Olean, on the label of certain snack foods such as potato chips and crackers. Olestra does not provide any calories because it is not digested or absorbed. Like sorbitol, this nondigestible characteristic may cause symptoms of gas, bloating, diarrhea, and abdominal pain. If you have these symptoms, check your diet for olestra content. You may need to reduce—or completely eliminate—your intake of foods that contain this product.

Insufficient Amount of Fiber and Water

Did you know that the average North American eats only half of the dietary fiber that he or she needs? Instead of eating the recommended

20 to 35 grams of fiber daily, most people consume just 10 to 15 grams. For people with constipation-prone irritable bowel, a low-fiber intake results in constipation and sometimes alternating constipation and diarrhea.

We wouldn't be surprised if you have tried a high-fiber diet in the past. You would be like the many people who come to our clinic convinced that fiber will not work or that they do not tolerate fiber. It makes perfect sense if you stopped a high-fiber diet when you found it didn't work or made you feel worse. However, you might have unknowingly fallen into the common pitfalls associated with trying a high-fiber diet without first seeking expert advice. Even some health care professionals, including physicians and dietitians, may have steered you wrong. Not all health care professionals understand the important intricacies of a high-fiber diet for constipation-prone irritable bowel.

The common reasons a high-fiber diet fails include:

- *Introducing a high-fiber diet too quickly.* Fiber should be introduced gradually, over three to four weeks, and more slowly with some people.
- *Insufficient fiber intake.* Some people think that if they eat whole wheat bread their diet is high in fiber. This is not so. Sometimes people eat lots of fiber some days, but little other days. To manage your symptoms effectively, a high-fiber intake is required daily.
- *The fibers that best regulate your bowel habit are not eaten in sufficient quantities.* Wheat-based fibers such as breakfast cereals with wheat bran, whole wheat bread, whole wheat crackers, and wheat bran muffins are the most effective in regulating your bowel habit.
- *The required amount of water is not consumed.* This is such a common mistake that we have come to expect it. We cannot make this point strongly enough: eight 8-ounce glasses of water are required daily for the fiber to work. Some people do not appreciate this on their first doctor visit and do not drink enough water. When their symptoms improve only marginally, we again stress the importance of water consumption. On follow-up visits, we find that the adequate water consumption, along with the high-fiber diet, has resulted in a regular bowel habit.

- *Some people do not like high-fiber foods.* Fiber can be an acquired taste. As such, it should be brought into a diet over a period of time on a graduated basis, for example, starting with 60 percent whole wheat bread, trying breakfast cereals made with whole wheat and combining this with a bran flake–type cereal, and trying muffins made with whole wheat flour. If you just don't think you can eat fiber-containing foods, we recommend a fiber supplement to control your symptoms.

Overcoming the Diet-Related Triggers of Irritable Bowel

Now that you understand which foods and habits trigger irritable bowel symptoms, we are going to review strategies to minimize these triggers and symptoms.

Eating Patterns

Change any eating patterns that are provoking your symptoms.

Eating Food Fast

Plan for a sufficient amount of time to eat. Make this a priority. Once you have prepared a meal, sit and try to relax while you eat. Sit for a few minutes after you finish. If you must eat while working at your desk, take at least ten to fifteen minutes to eat your food. Another strategy is to chew more per bite of food. This will slow down your intake and may result in you eating less because your brain has time to register when you've had enough to eat.

Eating Fast Food

You will feel best if you limit the fast food in your diet. The maximum number of times you should eat fast food is once per week, and once every two weeks if you note that your symptoms are particularly bad with fast food. Fast-food restaurants offer healthy food choices such as a grilled chicken breast sandwich, baked potatoes, tossed salad (which may be gas forming), and muffins. Try these for a change. Don't be misled into thinking all chicken and fish sandwiches are low in fat. Breaded and deep-fried chicken and fish sandwiches contain a lot of fat and therefore are likely not all that well tolerated. If you simply must have a burger, pass on the fries. French fries substantially increase the fat content of your meal, thus making it harder to digest.

Skipping Meals

To control your irritable bowel, it is important for you to eat three meals per day. You don't have to eat at precisely 7 A.M., noon, and 6 P.M., but you do need to eat something in the morning, the afternoon, and the evening. If you are concerned about weight gain, we are not suggesting that you eat large meals. Examples of balanced, low-calorie, nutritious meals that you are likely to tolerate include cereal, milk, and fruit, or a slice of toast and jam with a glass of juice in the morning; lunch could be a low-fat muffin and low-fat yogurt with a piece of fruit, or a sandwich of 1 to 2 ounces of a lean meat or cheese on whole wheat bread, and milk or low-fat yogurt; supper can be lean meat, fish, or chicken with rice or potato and vegetables, or pasta with a low-fat sauce (tomato or a cream sauce made with low-fat milk), and some vegetables.

If you are concerned about weight gain, watch your portion sizes. Portion distortion results in us eating the equivalent of many servings that we unknowingly count as one. Read food labels for the serving size and don't feel obligated to eat an entire portion served to you in a restaurant as many restaurants and fast-food outlets offer large portion sizes.

Keep in mind that eating small amounts throughout the day helps to curb your appetite. It also trains your body to burn off calories rather than storing them as fat, which is what happens if you eat one only meal per day.

Eating Junk Food

You don't need to give up junk food altogether. As with fast food, however, you will feel best if you keep your junk food intake to a minimum, perhaps once every one to two weeks. Also, you may need to decrease the amount of junk food you eat in a sitting if you tend to eat large amounts (a large bag of potato chips or cheese puffs at a time). Try to cut this to less than half or buy single-serving bags only. Low-fat snack foods that you might tolerate better are pretzels, low-fat potato snacks, rice cakes, and whole wheat crackers. Sweeter, low-fat snacks that you will likely tolerate are baby and digestive cookies, fig-date- or fruit-filled cookies, ginger snaps, breakfast cereal with milk (except cereals with nuts), granola bars without nuts, low-fat yogurt, and fruit canned in its own juice. (See pages 57 and 58 in chapter 5 for snacking ideas and the appendix for recipes.)

Overeating

Beware of occasions that promote overeating: for example, family and holiday celebrations, office parties, eating out, or eating your favorite meal. Once you have had enough to eat, stop. Whatever you didn't finish can be eaten later. For example, have dessert a few hours after your meal or save some of your main course for a snack later on. You will enjoy and tolerate foods much better if you follow this practice. To help avoid overeating, drink water before you start a meal; this helps make you feel full and reduces your likelihood of eating too much.

Symptom-Provoking Foods

Limit the symptom-provoking foods in your diet. If eaten occasionally, trigger foods may be tolerated in small amounts. However, we want to make it clear that it is important to follow your irritable bowel diet closely for at least the first six weeks. (Chapter 7 presents the different diets for irritable bowel.) If you don't follow the diet adjustments closely, you will not know whether the diet is effectively treating your symptoms. Once your symptoms are under control and you know how to treat them effectively, then you can experiment to see whether you tolerate certain trigger foods in small amounts, occasionally.

The Food Tolerance Test

It is important to make a clear distinction between food intolerance and food allergy. Food intolerance is just that—a food that your gut does not tolerate well. Your body produces symptoms in the process of digesting a food that it does not tolerate. We can develop food intolerances at any point in our lives. People often say to us, "I used to be able to eat anything—I had a cast-iron stomach. Now, I get these symptoms when I eat certain foods." Developing food intolerances is a common and natural phenomenon, especially as we age.

By contrast, food allergy results in a chemical response in your body, producing antibodies to a food that your body interprets as a foreign and potentially harmful substance. This process produces physical symptoms (see chapter 4 for more information on food allergy and intolerance). Food allergies are very rare, whereas food intolerances are very common. Irritable bowel symptoms are a result of food intolerance, not food allergy.

To test whether you tolerate a food, dietitians usually recommend a three-step process:

1. The first phase is to remove the food from your diet for a period of two to six weeks.
2. After two to six weeks, try a small to moderate amount of the food in question, preferably with a food you know that you tolerate, or by itself. Watch for symptoms you believe that the food causes. If you do not experience symptoms, it is likely that you tolerate the food, but it would be wise to test at another time to be sure.
3. If you experienced symptoms, put the food away for a week or more and try it again, in the same fashion—small amounts, with foods you know you tolerate, or by itself. If on the third try of a particular food you experience symptoms, then you do not tolerate the food. If you want to feel better, you should probably remove the food from your diet.

On occasions when you plan to enjoy a trigger food (after your symptoms are under control), eat a small- to moderate-sized portion and try not to have any other trigger foods with it or earlier in the day. For example, if you know that you are going to have a salad (a gassy food) with supper, don't eat trigger foods at noon. Doing so will increase the likelihood that you will not tolerate the food that you are planning to enjoy at night. Strategies like this will keep your symptoms to a minimum.

If you plan to eat trigger foods over a period of time, such as over a holiday season, don't neglect consuming enough fiber (primarily if you are constipation prone) and water, consistently. This should minimize the effects of trigger foods. So when you deviate from your diet, don't let it all go. You will want to feel well enough to enjoy the celebration.

Insufficient Amount of Fiber and Water

Increase the amount of fiber in your diet. People who have constipation-prone irritable bowel will need an increased-fiber diet. People with an alternating bowel habit may require more than the standard 10 to 15 grams of fiber consumed by the average North American, but less than a person with constipation-prone irritable bowel. The next chapter will help you sort out the amount of fiber you require.

The amount of fiber recommended for the average North American is between 20 and 35 grams per day. The amount you need depends on the severity of your constipation. For example, if you have long-lasting constipation and have difficulty moving your bowels once per week, your needs will be in the higher range, likely 25 to 35 grams per day. However, if you have constipation for two or three days, followed by loose stools for several days, your needs may be in the 15- to 20-gram range. Chapter 7 contains additional guidelines on how to increase your fiber intake.

Food and Symptom Record

Now that you know the common nutrition-related causes of irritable bowel, it is time to discover the specific eating patterns, behaviors, or trigger foods that may be causing your symptoms. To do this we recommend that you use the food and symptom record on pages 80 and 81.

For one week, you need to document the foods you eat and the symptoms you experience. At the end of the week, you should study your record to uncover the connections between the foods you ate or your eating patterns and the symptoms you experienced.

A food and symptom record is an important step in getting control over your symptoms. We highly recommend that you don't skip it. It's the most useful tool for looking at your diet and symptoms and determining the relationship between the two. If you don't keep a record, you might not appreciate that you have some symptom-provoking habits or that you eat some symptom-provoking foods. It is like trying to drive with your eyes covered.

How to Complete a Food and Symptom Record

We recommend that you record the six following irritable bowel symptoms, if and when you experience them over a one-week period. Record the severity of your symptoms from 1 (minimal/negligible) to 10 (extreme severity):

- Abdominal pain
- Constipation
- Diarrhea
- Gas
- Bloating
- Heartburn (not an irritable bowel symptom, but associated with irritable bowel)

Be sure to record both the foods you eat and the symptoms you experience. This is important because the specific diet adjustments that we recommend in chapter 7 are based on specific sets of symptoms. Each person who has irritable bowel is unique. The type and severity of symptoms differ from person to person. If you do not have a problem with gas and bloating or diarrhea, there is no need to follow the diet guidelines that are designed to control these symptoms.

The following recommendations will help you to keep track of your meals, snacks, and symptoms:

- For greatest accuracy, make your entries throughout the day just after you eat or experience symptoms. If you are unable to do this, try to make your notes at the end of each day.
- Note all food and beverages consumed.
- Record the amount of food or beverage consumed; for example, 8 ounces of skim milk or orange juice, a large potato, or one small chicken breast with the skin removed.

- Write down how the food was prepared; for example, whether the chicken was fried or baked or you used 1 teaspoon of oil.
- In the section labeled "Water," record the number of 8-ounce glasses of water you consumed that day.
- You will find your record easier to analyze if you write the foods in blue and the symptoms in red next to the foods you suspect provoked your symptoms.

How to Analyze Your Food and Symptom Record

The next important step is to analyze your food and symptom record for foods and habits that may be triggering your symptoms. The food-symptom connections that you will identify through this record will tell you where to concentrate your dietary efforts to manage your irritable bowel symptoms. We recommend that you make a list of the foods and eating patterns that you singled out as causing your symptoms, as well as a separate list of the irritable bowel symptoms you experienced.

Look at Your Eating Patterns

Did you eat fast food or junk food? Did you overeat? Did you skip any meals or eat a lot one day and little the next? Do you remember eating quickly or on the run? Were you stressed? It might be easiest to answer each of these questions separately while analyzing your record for symptoms you may have experienced as a result. See "Matching Symptoms to Healthy Eating Adjustments" on page 84 for the symptoms you may experience as a result of each eating pattern.

Analyze Your Record for Any Symptom-Provoking Foods

If you are unsure which foods are gassy, fatty, or spicy, the eating guidelines in chapter 7 provide tips on reducing gassy, fatty, and spicy foods. Remember, the amount of a trigger food is important as well as whether you ate one or more trigger foods at a sitting. A combination of trigger foods might result in symptoms, but any one of them eaten alone might not. Whether you ate trigger foods throughout the day or some the day before is relevant and may make your symptoms worse. How much soft drink or juice did you drink daily?

FOOD AND SYMPTOM RECORD

Sample Day	Monday	Tuesday	Wednesday
Water: 8 cups	Water	Water	Water
Breakfast 7 A.M. ¹/₂ cup All Bran cereal; 1 cup low-fat milk; 6 oz. orange juice; 6 oz. tea			
Lunch 12:30 P.M. Sandwich on whole wheat bread: 2 oz. chicken, 2 tsp. mayo, lettuce, and tomato; 1 cup french fries; 1 cup low-fat milk *Symptoms: about 1:30 P.M.— abdominal pain, gas, diarrhea*			
Snack 4:30 P.M. Small wheat bran muffin; 6 oz. tea			
Dinner 6:30 P.M. Oven-grilled pork chop, 4 oz., fat removed; 1 cup mashed potatoes; ¹/₂ cup steamed broccoli; ¹/₂ cup cooked carrots *Symptoms: just after supper— gas and bloating*			
Snack 8:30 P.M. Potato chips, 1 oz. bag, 1 can cola *Symptoms: 9 P.M.—gas and bloating*			

Thursday		Friday		Saturday		Sunday	
Water		Water		Water		Water	

Review Your Record for Fiber and Water Content

Did you eat whole wheat bread most of the time? Did you eat wheat bran cereals? How often? Did you choose whole wheat crackers or wheat bran muffins? How much water did you drink? How many 8-ounce glasses per day? On how many days, if any, did you drink eight 8-ounce glasses? Analyzing the food record for fiber content is particularly important for people with constipation-prone or alternating constipation and diarrhea irritable bowel. See "Fiber Content of Selected Foods" in chapter 7.

Analyze Why You Eat the Foods You Eat

Many people struggle to control what they eat even after they know which foods cause irritable bowel symptoms. This is where nutrition and psychological factors are mixed. There are two types of psychological issues that are common here. The first is general lifestyle and emotional stress-related issues. The lifestyle issue is related to a very active, busy lifestyle in which we juggle many demands. As such, finding time to eat can be a challenge. People pressed for time will often eat on the run and choose fast foods or unhealthy prepared foods. You might discover that some foods you choose that aggravate your irritable bowel are a result of your lifestyle. If so, we recommend that you read chapter 9 on stress management and chapter 11 on readiness for change.

The second type of psychological issue is eating when under stress. Many people report that they eat when they are upset or under stress. Usually, it is unhealthy foods that people turn to during such situations. So, when analyzing your food record, ask yourself if any of the foods you eat that trigger your irritable bowel symptoms are related to stress issues in your life. If they are, chapter 9 might be very helpful to you.

7

Healthy Eating Adjustments for Specific Symptoms

Before diving into this chapter, we strongly recommend that you first read chapters 5 and 6 if you haven't done so yet. They contain important tips for adopting a healthy diet as well as insights into how certain eating habits and food choices can provoke irritable bowel symptoms. Nutrition adjustment is an essential component of treating irritable bowel. And in our experience, nutrition management of irritable bowel symptoms is most often very effective for reducing symptoms.

In this chapter, we offer specific diet adjustments and practical nutrition guidelines that have proven in our clinic and in research studies to be very effective at relieving irritable bowel symptoms. There's a lot to learn, so you may want to read this chapter more than once. It could prove difficult to digest, so to speak, in one reading.

The following table previews the recommended diet adjustments for the six most common symptoms associated with irritable bowel. In the following pages, we will explain each of these adjustments and show how they can work together if you experience more than one symptom at a time.

MATCHING SYMPTOMS TO HEALTHY EATING ADJUSTMENTS

Irritable Bowel Symptom	Eating Adjustment
Abdominal pain	High fiber
	Low gassy foods
	Low caffeine
	Low fat
Constipation	High fiber
	Low caffeine
Diarrhea	Low caffeine
	Low fat and low spice
Gas	Low gassy foods
	Low caffeine
Bloating	Low gassy foods
	High fiber
Heartburn (technically, heartburn is not an irritable bowel symptom, but it is common with irritable bowel)	Antireflux

Abdominal Pain

Abdominal pain is associated with a number of other symptoms. Pain is related to constipation or diarrhea or to the sensation that gases are being trapped in the intestines. Irritable bowel may react with abdominal pain to caffeine intake or high-fat foods that are hard to digest. Based on the four potential nutrition-related causes, there are four potential diet adjustments to consider that minimize abdominal pain.

Fiber can help if your pain symptoms are related to constipation or to alternating constipation and diarrhea. If abdominal pain is due to gas, then a low gassy foods diet relieves discomfort caused by gas-producing foods. Caffeine may cause stomach pain; therefore, limiting caffeine will result in less pain. High-fat foods are hard to digest and may cause discomfort or abdominal cramping when the gut revs up to digest these foods. Thus, limiting fat in the diet will reduce pain resulting from digesting fatty foods.

Abdominal pain is commonly treated with a high-fiber diet (for people who are constipation prone or who have alternating constipation and diarrhea), combined with a diet low in gassy foods. In fact, this diet combination is recommended most in our clinic. Also, if you have spasms or intense shooting pain in your bowel, a high-fiber diet will likely benefit you. However, you will need to add fiber to your diet very gradually. You may also need to talk with your doctor about medication to treat this type of pain. Refer to chapter 10 for more information on managing the pain associated with irritable bowel.

Constipation

The next major symptom, constipation, is primarily treated with a high-fiber diet. Fiber is recommended because it is a water-attracting substance and therefore holds water in the stool, making it softer and easier to pass. When a person is constipated, fiber also speeds up the rate stools move through the large bowel.

Even though fiber can relieve constipation, not every high-fiber diet is appropriate for someone with irritable bowel. A typical high-fiber diet needs to be modified to remove certain fibers that may be poorly tolerated. We often recommend removing certain fruits and vegetables, dried peas and beans, and nuts and seeds. These foods contain gas-producing fibers that can cause more discomfort from gas than discomfort caused by constipation. We often recommend the high-fiber, low gassy foods diet combination mentioned earlier to treat constipation because people with irritable bowel who are constipated tend to also have problems with gas and bloating. The high-fiber diet in this book is designed specifically for people with irritable bowel who are experiencing constipation or alternating constipation and diarrhea (see page 89).

Diarrhea

Diarrhea may be relieved by reducing or eliminating caffeine in your diet. Caffeine has been found to be a major cause of diarrhea for a significant number of people with irritable bowel. Caffeine is a stimulant, and people who have diarrhea do not need more bowel stimulation. Sometimes caffeine must be limited or avoided.

Fatty or spicy foods can also cause diarrhea. You may have experienced this yourself on occasion. It is wise to limit fat and spice in your diet if you find that you experience diarrhea after eating spicy and fatty foods. This may mean reducing the amount of fat and spice you cook with and/or decreasing the number of times you eat fatty or spicy foods. Chocolate, which contains a drug like caffeine and is high in fat, has also been linked to diarrhea.

Research shows that people with a diarrhea-prone irritable bowel may get symptom relief from an exclusion diet (besides diarrhea, the symptoms that may decrease when you are on an exclusion diet include abdominal pain, bloating, and gas). A common exclusion diet allows all meat (except beef) and fish. Dairy products are replaced with soy products. Cereals such as wheat and oats are eliminated, but rice is allowed. Other common restrictions are yeast, citrus, caffeinated drinks, and tap water. If you have diarrhea-prone irritable bowel and want to try an exclusion diet, we strongly advise you to work with a medical or nutrition professional. Exclusion diets are restrictive and may result in nutritional deficiencies.

We do not recommend a high-fiber diet for people with diarrhea. In our experience, people with diarrhea do not commonly benefit from eating more fiber. There are exceptions to every rule, however. Many people with diarrhea-prone irritable bowel have episodes where their bowels can be constipated. Increasing fiber in the diet can sometimes help diarrhea because the liquid-holding properties of the fiber absorb the excess fluid in the gut and help to slow down the rapid movement of the liquid stool.

Gas and Bloating

Gas is a common problem that causes bloating and abdominal pain when it cannot be expelled. In addition, producing and passing a lot of gas can make social situations uncomfortable. Therefore, a low gassy foods diet is appropriate when dealing with this symptom.

Gas can also come from swallowing air. When you eat quickly or gulp foods, you may draw air into your digestive tract. We have also observed that some people have a lot of gas production when they drink coffee. We are uncertain of the reason for the gas production—perhaps the stimulant effects of caffeine—but the low-caffeine guidelines might be worth trying for a couple of weeks to see if it does help (see "The Food Tolerance Test" in chapter 6).

Bloating seems to be the most difficult symptom to treat. It may be linked to constipation or eating gassy foods. It is treated with a high-fiber diet (for people with constipation and alternating constipation and diarrhea) and a low gassy foods diet. Often, people who do not pass stools for two or more days feel bloated; a high-fiber diet will result in more frequent bowel motions. You will need to increase fiber gradually. (We will discuss fiber later in the chapter.) Fiber also helps to remove gassy foods from the diet that contribute to the bloating. People who are prone to diarrhea may also experience bloating and will get relief by removing gassy foods from their diet.

Heartburn

Heartburn is not a true symptom of irritable bowel, but it is associated with it. We include this symptom and the diet adjustment to correct it because in our experience a significant number of people with irritable bowel suffer from heartburn. Coffee drinkers are also more likely to experience heartburn owing to the caffeine. Fortunately, heartburn is very amenable to diet adjustments.

Heartburn is caused by the underlying motility disorder associated with an irritable bowel. Because the digestive tract moves food along in a disordered manner, foods reflux (go in reverse) from the stomach back up the esophagus. Stomach acids in the food cause the esophagus to feel like it is on fire or burning. There are other reasons for heartburn, such as a hiatal hernia, which may cause you to reflux stomach contents, but the nutrition treatment is the same: an antireflux diet.

The antireflux diet removes foods that would otherwise cause the muscle at the bottom of the esophagus to weaken, allowing more foods to reflux and cause heartburn. The antireflux diet also removes acidic-type foods that people with reflux problems tend to tolerate poorly. When people with heartburn follow this diet, the results are usually dramatic. Even people who require medication to get their symptoms under control can be weaned off drugs once they have been on an antireflux diet for six to eight weeks.

Where Should You Start?

Very rarely does a person need to follow all six diet adjustments. We recommend that you choose your eating strategy based on your particular symptoms. Plan to start with just one or two diet adjustments. Three or four diet adjustments may benefit you, but tackling that many diet adjustments at the same time is usually too much to manage. Remember, there is no set formula for someone with irritable bowel to follow. You must figure out for yourself the factors that cause your symptoms. By starting out with one or two diet adjustments and gradually adding another diet modification (if you believe you need another based on your symptoms), you are more able to determine which changes are most helpful to you.

For people with constipation-prone irritable bowel or alternating constipation and diarrhea, we suggest starting with the high-fiber diet. We recommend between 20 and 35 grams of fiber daily. If gas and bloating are significant symptoms, then we suggest that you also try the low gassy foods diet at the outset. We suggest that you try both of these together because you will likely experience dramatic symptom relief. If initially you try the high-fiber diet alone, you might have less effective results.

Your symptoms will tell you whether you need to introduce any other diet adjustments. The timing of diet introduction depends on two factors: the severity of a particular symptom and how many diet adjustments you feel that you can manage at the same time. For example, if you have abdominal pain and have become aware that caffeine and excessive gas production are causing this symptom, you can start to gradually reduce your caffeine intake. You might also get relief by simultaneously following the low gassy foods diet. If you are constipated and are experiencing heartburn but have little gas and bloating, you might want to start a high-fiber diet first and introduce an antireflux diet a bit later, if your symptoms of heartburn are not too severe.

There is flexibility on how you introduce diet adjustments. You choose which eating strategy to start with and whether or when you introduce any more strategies. You are in control of managing your symptoms. Be sure to try each diet adjustment for at least six weeks. This allows sufficient time for you to become adjusted to the diet and to evaluate its effectiveness.

The Diet Adjustments

This section contains the diet adjustments that will help to reduce or eliminate your symptoms of irritable bowel.

The High-Fiber Diet: The Basic Factor

It takes 20 to 35 grams of fiber per day to treat constipation or alternating constipation and diarrhea. The amount you need depends on whether you have an alternating bowel habit, or on the severity of your constipation. Generally, your needs will be in the lower recommended range if you have an alternating bowel habit, and you will probably have to introduce fiber more gradually. If you have severe constipation, such as your bowels moving less than once every five days, you will need to be in the higher range of the recommended fiber intake.

For a high-fiber diet to work, you will need to:

- Eat the most effective type of fiber
- Eat a sufficient amount of fiber
- Eat a high-fiber diet every day
- Drink plenty of water and other caffeine-free liquids daily

You Need the Most Effective Type of Fiber

You may know that dietary fiber is found in whole grain products, fruits, vegetables, and meat alternates such as nuts and dried peas and beans. These four food groups contain different types of fiber.

Fiber is classified into two main types: soluble and insoluble. Most of these foods contain a mixture of fibers; however, some foods are known for the specific type of fiber they contain. For example, whole wheat products and some vegetables such as broccoli and carrots contain primarily insoluble fiber, while fruits, dried peas and beans, some vegetables, and oats are known for their soluble fiber content. Soluble fiber has a cholesterol-lowering effect in your body. Also, this type of fiber helps people with diabetes control their blood sugar.

The insoluble fiber found in whole grain wheat products is the most effective in regulating your bowel habit. Good sources of this fiber are whole wheat bread, whole wheat crackers, wheat bran muffins, and breakfast cereals containing wheat bran. Insoluble fiber found in whole wheat products is the fiber of choice for the high-fiber diet.

As mentioned earlier, we often recommend avoiding certain fruits and vegetables, dried peas and beans, and nuts and seeds because the fibers in these foods produce excessive gas and worsen irritable bowel symptoms. Also, the fibers found in these foods are not as effective as wheat in regulating bowel habits. Guidelines on how to remove these foods from your diet start on page 95.

It is very common for people who first come to our clinic to have tried a high-fiber diet in which they consumed a lot of fiber from a variety of sources. They report that they felt excessively gassy and bloated and that there was little change in their bowel habit. Usually, these people were choosing fibers from fruits, vegetables, and dried beans. Once we advised them to focus on wheat-based fiber and avoid fiber that causes unreasonable amounts of gas production, their bowel habit improved and their bloating and abdominal pain decreased.

The high-fiber diet recommended here focuses on wheat-based fiber. The fiber found in oatmeal and oat bran is not as effective as wheat in treating bowel habits. People with irritable bowel tolerate oatmeal and oat bran fine, but these sources of fiber will not help to regulate their bowel habit. However, wheat bran may be added to oatmeal (and other hot or cold cereals) to improve the amount and quality of fiber and to regulate your bowel habit.

If you have a problem with gas and bloating and you are on a high-fiber diet, you should not eat multigrain breads, crackers, or bagels because multigrain products may have sesame, poppy, flax, and sunflower seeds, which will probably make you feel gassy. If you want fiber but have a problem with gas and bloating, you should eat bread and crackers that are wheat bran– or whole wheat–based.

You Need to Eat a Sufficient Amount of Fiber

A common mistake people make when they start a high-fiber diet is that they simply eat whole wheat bread and figure their diet is high in fiber. Not so. There is more to a high-fiber diet than whole wheat bread. Remember, you need to consume 20 to 35 grams of fiber per day. We will show you how to achieve this high-fiber intake with practical and easy-to-understand guidelines (see page 92).

People often ask if it is possible to eat too much fiber. It is. A fiber intake of more than 35 grams per day is too much for most people with irritable bowel. If you consume more than this, you will likely experience discomfort in your belly and feel very bloated. Consuming more than 50 grams per day may decrease your body's ability to absorb some nutrients, such as iron, zinc, magnesium, and calcium.

You Need to Eat a High-Fiber Diet Every Day

A high-fiber diet needs to be followed seven days a week. Feel free to change some of your routine on weekends (sleep in, have brunch instead of breakfast and lunch), but you must eat that fiber.

You Need to Drink Plenty of Water and Other Caffeine-Free Liquids Every Day

This guideline is every bit as important as the first three. Fiber and water work very well together to regulate bowel movements, but neither works well by itself. As noted earlier, not getting enough water is likely the leading reason why high-fiber diets fail.

Drinking eight 8-ounce glasses of water each day can be a bit intimidating to some. As with anything you embark on, it becomes much easier once you get into the habit. It also helps to plan ahead. Many patients in our clinic are successful when they drink two 8-ounce glasses of water with each meal. This means that six of the eight 8-ounce glasses of water are consumed at mealtimes alone. Drinking water with your meals also helps prevent overeating and facilitates the mixing of fiber and fluid in the digestive tract. Another option, whether you work outside the home or not, is to drink water throughout the day from a large container. Try to drink the equivalent of three 8-ounce glasses of water by lunch, and another three by the end of the afternoon. This makes six—you need to drink only two more.

If you take fiber in the form of a bulking agent such as Metamucil, you will be drinking one glass of water each time you take a serving. The manufacturer also recommends that you drink a second glass of water with each dose. If you take Metamucil twice daily, this represents half the water intake you need. However, if you divide your normal dose of Metamucil into three, you would be taking six 8-ounce glasses of water per day, or 75 percent of the water that you need.

Whatever scheme works for you, it is best to spread the water intake throughout the day and not leave it all to be consumed in the evening. We generally tell people that 25 percent of the water requirement, or two 8-ounce glasses per day, may come from caffeine-free sources other than water, such as juice, water, milk, herbal tea, or noncola soft drinks. You may drink more of these liquids if you like, but count only two glasses for your daily water intake.

Making the Most of a High-Fiber Diet

For a high-fiber diet to be most effective, you should practice each of the following steps:

1. *Choose wheat-based whole grain products:*
   - Whole wheat bread
   - Wheat bran bread
   - Whole wheat crackers
   - Wheat bran muffins
   - Whole wheat cereal
2. *Choose one concentrated source of fiber daily* (it is important to introduce fiber gradually; see the list on page 94):
   - A very-high-fiber cereal such as All Bran, 100% Bran, Bran Buds with Psyllium, or Fiber One
   - Natural bran
   - A bulking agent, such as Metamucil or Prodiem
3. *Drink eight or more 8-ounce glasses of water daily.* Caffeine-free liquids such as juice, milk, herbal tea, and noncola soft drinks can be counted as two of the eight glasses of water per day.

These high-fiber guidelines are designed to treat constipation or alternating constipation and diarrhea. To get the most fiber, check the fiber content on the food label and look for descriptors such as "high fiber," "good source," "more fiber," or "added fiber," and select the item with the highest fiber content.

FIBER CONTENT ACCORDING TO THE FOOD LABEL

Description on Label	Translation
High fiber	5 grams or more per serving
Good source	2.5–4.9 grams per serving
More or added fiber	At least 2.5 grams or more per serving (compared to a standard serving size of the conventional food)

Also, check bread labels for the term *whole wheat*. Breads with this term must be made from 100 percent whole wheat flour. By contrast, wheat bread may contain some white flour and some whole wheat flour. Check the ingredient list and buy the bread that contains the most whole wheat flour.

Beyond choosing to eat whole wheat products, we also recommend that you eat a concentrated source of fiber each day. As the guidelines on fiber content note, there are several options for concentrated sources of fiber:

- Very-high-fiber cereals provide 10 or more grams of fiber per ½ cup. They should be substituted only with a cereal of a similar fiber content.
- Natural bran, also called baker's bran, looks a bit like sawdust. Besides being used in baking, it can be added to cereal and other foods to increase their fiber content.
- Bulking agents, such as Metamucil or Prodiem, are made from natural plant fibers and are safe to take. They are not stimulant laxatives, and your bowels will not become dependent on them.

If you have never been a cereal eater, a bulking agent may suit you better than a very-high-fiber cereal. Maybe you would prefer to add natural bran to foods that you eat throughout the day. For variety, you may alternate your choice of a concentrated source of fiber from day to day. Gradually introducing a concentrated source of fiber is recommended because it might otherwise cause discomfort in the abdomen.

Introducing a concentrated fiber source includes:

- Very-high-fiber cereal: All Bran, 100% Bran, Bran Buds with Psyllium, Fiber One. Start with ¼ cup per day for seven to ten days, then increase to ½ cup daily. You may combine the very-high-fiber cereal with a lower-fiber cereal of your choice; for example, ½ cup of All Bran mixed with ½ cup of your favorite cereal.
- Natural bran: Start with 2 tablespoons per day for seven to ten days, then increase to 4 tablespoons daily. Add to cereals, casseroles, stews, baked goods, or whatever you like.
- Bulking agent: Metamucil, Normacol, Prodiem. Start with 1 rounded (not heaping, not level) teaspoon each day for seven days, then increase by adding another teaspoon at another time of day for seven more days. If you are using sugar-free Metamucil, 1 rounded teaspoon is recommended; if you are using regular Metamucil (which contains sugar), use 1 level tablespoon. You might need to add another teaspoon, preferably at a different time of day (1 teaspoon, three times per day), or double one dose (2 rounded teaspoons at one time, 1 teaspoon at another). You should not have to exceed a total of 4 rounded teaspoons per day.

You might need to introduce the concentrated source of fiber more slowly, especially if you have alternating constipation and diarrhea and/or frequent and intense abdominal pain. If you have these symptoms, start with half of the amount suggested, and increase by half of the amount in the times allotted. For example, start with ½ teaspoon of a bulking agent per day and increase by ½ teaspoon each week, instead of starting with 1 teaspoon daily and increasing by 1 teaspoon. Results might take longer, but you will tolerate the fiber better.

The final step in successfully adopting a high-fiber diet is to drink eight or more 8-ounce glasses of water each day. If you skip this, the high-fiber diet will not work. Many people make great efforts to increase the fiber in their diet, but they do not consume enough water, which turns out to be the only reason that their bowel function does not improve satisfactorily. When they get the recommended amount of water, though, they get results: a regular bowel habit and significant symptom relief.

It takes time for a high-fiber diet to start working, so it is wise to not expect results before the first two or three weeks. Your bowel is irritable! This means it might object to diet changes even if these changes will improve symptoms over the long run.

If you follow the high-fiber diet as advised—eating the recommended amount and type of fiber daily and drinking eight 8-ounce glasses of water daily—and your bowel movements are better but not as regular as you would like, you may want to increase your concentrated source of fiber a bit more. For example, you may want to add another ¼ to ½ cup of cereal in the afternoon; take 1 to 2 rounded teaspoons of a bulking agent; or add 1 to 2 tablespoons of natural bran at a different time of day from when you ate your first concentrated source of fiber. You may need this extra-concentrated source of fiber only every other day. As always, make sure that you have at least eight 8-ounce glasses of water daily.

The Low Gassy Foods Diet: Go Farther on Less Gas

A high-fiber diet is often teamed with a low gassy foods diet to ease a number of irritable bowel symptoms. Reducing the number of gassy foods in your diet will help to treat the symptoms of abdominal pain, gas, and bloating.

Certain foods are gassy because they contain carbohydrates, a form of sugar, that is not completely digested in the small bowel. When these sugars get to the large bowel, lots of bacteria digest them, producing gas in the process. This is what makes you feel gassy, bloated, and in pain. Certain fruits and vegetables and dried beans and peas may make you feel particularly gassy and bloated. This is because these foods contain the carbohydrates that are usually not totally broken down in the small bowel. Soft drinks also increase intestinal gas as the air bubbles in the soda enter your digestive system and cause you to feel gassy.

It is common for bloating to become worse as the day progresses. Some people say they practically need clothing a size larger by the evening! Fortunately, cutting down on gassy foods will bring relief to your bloating-type symptoms.

FIBER CONTENT OF SELECTED FOODS

Food Portion Size	Dietary Fiber (g)	Food Portion Size	Dietary Fiber (g)
Grain Products		Filberts, shelled, dried,	
Brown rice, long grain,		unblanched, 10 nuts	0.9
cooked, 1/2 cup	1.5	Peanut butter, chunky,	
Cracked wheat bread, 1 slice	1.3	2 tablespoons	2.2
Cream of wheat, cooked,		Peanut butter, smooth,	
1 cup	0.9	2 tablespoons	1.8
Light rye bread, 1 slice	1.6	Peanuts, shelled, dry	
Multigrain bread, 1 slice	1.6	roasted, raw, 10 nuts	0.7
Natural bran/baker's bran,		*Fruits*	
2 tablespoons	3.0	Apple, fresh with skin,	
Oat bran, cooked, 1 cup	0.9	1 medium	2.6
Rolled oats, cooked, 1 cup	4.2	Apple, fresh without skin,	
Wheat bran bread, 1 slice	2.1	1 medium	2.4
Wheat bran muffin,		Applesauce, 1/2 cup	1.5
1 medium	3.8	Apricots, dried, uncooked,	
White noodles, cooked,		5 halves	1.4
1/2 cup	1.1	Banana, 1 medium	2.0
White rice, long grain,		Blueberries, fresh, 1/2 cup	2.0
cooked, 1/2 cup	0.4	Cantaloupe, 1/4 whole	0.9
Whole wheat bread, 1 slice	1.7	Cherries, sweet, 10	0.7
Whole wheat noodles,		Dates, 3	0.7
cooked, 1 cup	2.3	Grapefruit, 1/2	0.8
		Grapes with skin, 1 cup	0.8
Legumes		Orange, 1 medium	2.4
Baked beans, 1/2 cup	9.9	Papaya, 1 medium	5.3
Dried peas, cooked, 1/2 cup	2.9	Peach, fresh, 1 medium	
Kidney beans, 1/2 cup	7.9	with skin	1.6
Lentils, cooked, 1/2 cup	4.3	Pear, fresh, 1 medium	
Navy beans, cooked, 1/2 cup	6.3	with skin	5.0
		Pineapple, 1/2 cup	0.9
Nuts		Plums, 5 damson	5.3
Almonds, dry roasted,		Prunes, 3	1.8
unblanched, 10 nuts	1.6		

Food Portion Size	Dietary Fiber (g)	Food Portion Size	Dietary Fiber (g)
Raisins, ¼ cup	2.5	Corn, 1 ear	6.6
Raspberries, ½ cup	3.0	Onions, raw, diced, ½ cup	1.0
Rhubarb, cooked, ½ cup	1.7	Parsnip, cooked, ½ cup	3.1
Strawberries, 1 cup	3.0	Peas, green, cooked, ½ cup	3.6
Vegetables		Potatoes, baked, 1 medium	4.5
Asparagus, cooked, 4 spears	1.0	Potatoes, boiled, 1 medium	4.0
Bean sprouts (mung), raw, ½ cup	0.6	Spinach, cooked, ½ cup	2.1
		Spinach, raw, 1 cup	1.5
Beans, green or yellow, cooked, ½ cup	1.5	Squash, winter, all varieties, baked, ½ cup	2.9
Beans, lima, cooked, ½ cup	4.3	Squash, summer, all varieties, boiled, ½ cup	1.5
Broccoli, cooked, ½ cup	1.9		
Brussels sprouts, cooked, ½ cup	3.4	Sweet potato, baked with skin, ½ medium	1.7
Cabbage, cooked, ½ cup	1.3	Sweet potato, baked without skin, ½ medium	1.7
Carrots, cooked, ½ cup	2.1		
Carrots, raw, 1 medium	2.0	Sweet potato, candied, 1 piece	2.3
Cauliflower, cooked, ½ cup	1.0		
Celery, raw, diced, ½ cup	0.9	Tomato, raw, 1 medium	1.5
Corn, cooked, ½ cup	3.0	Turnip, cooked, ½ cup	2.3

Source: Health Canada, Canadian Nutrient File, 2005, www.healthcanada.ca/cnf.

Pay Attention to How You Are Eating

- Try to avoid gulping foods or eating quickly, because you swallow more air when you eat like this, which may increase intestinal gas.
- Try not to skip meals. Skipping meals encourages the gastrointestinal tract to fill with air.
- Avoid chewing gum or sucking on hard candy, which introduces a lot of air into the gastrointestinal tract.
- Avoid using a straw to drink liquids. More air is swallowed using straws.

Pay Attention to What You Are Eating

Certain foods are gas forming. For at least the six-week trial period, avoid:

- All raw vegetables, including salads.
- The following vegetables, even if they are cooked:

Broccoli	Pimentos
Brussels sprouts	Radishes
Cabbage	Red and green peppers
Cauliflower	Rutabaga
Corn	Sauerkraut
Cucumbers	Scallions
Kohlrabi	Shallots
Leek	Turnips
Onions	

- Dried peas and beans, including:

Black-eyed peas	Lima beans
Kidney beans	Navy beans
Lentils	Split peas

- The following fruits:

Apples, unpeeled	Honeydew melon
Avocados	Prunes
Cantaloupe	Watermelon

- Miscellaneous foods, including:

Beer	Popcorn
Grits	Seeds
Hard-boiled eggs	Soft drinks
Nuts	Wheat germ

Choose the Following Foods

Better choices of foods include:

- Cooked vegetables such as:

Asparagus	Carrots
Beets	Green beans

Green peas	Squash
Mushrooms	Sweet potatoes
Potatoes	Yellow beans
Pumpkin	Zucchini
Spinach	

- The following fruits:

Apples, peeled	Nectarines, ripe
Bananas, soft, ripe	Oranges
Fruit, canned	Peaches, ripe
Grapefruit	Pears, ripe
Kiwis	

In looking over the low gassy foods guidelines, you likely noticed the large number of fruits, vegetables, and other foods that should be limited or avoided. Although these foods are otherwise healthy, they are not tolerated very well by people with irritable bowel who have gas and bloating as significant symptoms. Fortunately, there are nutritious fruits and vegetables that are known to be less gassy. To minimize their gas-producing qualities, vegetables should be cooked and fruit canned or eaten ripe (when the fruit and skin are soft). Some people report that bananas cause stomach pain. If you find that any of the suggested fruits and vegetables bother you, you should avoid them.

Because the low gassy foods diet restricts many fruits and vegetables, the produce that you do eat should provide optimum nutrition. Some of the most important nutrients to obtain are beta carotene or vitamin A, vitamin C, and folate.

Carotenoids, particularly beta carotene, which changes into vitamin A, perform many functions in your overall health. Plus, as an antioxidant, vitamin A may offer protection from some diseases and aspects of aging. Vitamin C is another antioxidant vitamin that protects the body much the same way as vitamin A. Among many other responsibilities, vitamin C helps form the connective tissue that holds the many structures of the body together. It also keeps capillaries and gums healthy and helps the body to absorb iron from plant sources.

Folate is particularly important for all women of child-bearing age. Pregnant women who do not get enough folic acid (folate), especially during the first trimester, have a greater risk of delivering a baby with neural tube defects such as spina bifida. In the United States, enriched flour is fortified with folate. This means that the baked products and pasta that you buy (with enriched flour written on the label) or the enriched flour you use in baking will be fortified with folate. If you eat six servings of enriched grain products daily, you will have 80 percent of the folate that you require. The level of folate fortification varies among different countries; for example, in Canada enriched flour is fortified with less folate than in the United States and is designed to increase the folate content of an eighteen- to thirty-four-year-old woman by 50 percent. Women of child-bearing age living in Canada need to ensure that they choose foods high in folate on a regular basis.

The following foods are generally well tolerated by those with irritable bowel. Try to choose these foods as often as you can. Remember, the vegetables will need to be cooked.

WELL-TOLERATED NUTRIENT POWERHOUSES

Vitamin A	Vitamin C	Folate
Carrots	Oranges/orange juice	Oranges/orange juice
Spinach	Spinach	Spinach
Sweet potatoes	Grapefruit/grapefruit juice	Wheat germ
Winter squash	Tomatoes/tomato juice	Asparagus
Pumpkin	Baked potato with skin	Avocadoes

As you can see, some foods are high in more than one nutrient. For example, orange juice is high in vitamin C and folate, and spinach is high in all three nutrients.

If you are following a low gassy foods diet, there are circumstances when a multivitamin/mineral supplement is suggested:

- If you do not like or regularly eat the foods that contain significant amounts of vitamins A and C and folate.
- If you are also following an antireflux diet. The antireflux diet removes tomatoes and citrus fruits from your diet (see page 107).

If you feel less gassy and bloated at the end of the usual six-week trial period, we suggest you add in the foods that you missed the most—in small amounts and occasionally. For example, if you miss broccoli, try a small to moderate amount at a meal (see the section on food tolerance in chapter 6). If you really missed eating salads, try a small side salad with foods that you know you tolerate. Note that certain foods might always provoke symptoms no matter how little or how infrequently you eat them.

It's best to keep your intake of any gassy foods to small- to moderate-sized servings, two or three times a week. If you reintroduce gassy foods and eat them as often as you previously did, then you will likely feel as you did before you started the low-gassy foods diet.

If the low gassy foods diet does not significantly relieve the gas and bloating in six weeks, the restrictions are not working and you should discontinue the diet.

By choice or mistake, you are bound to eat foods that will make your symptoms worse. People often worry that they are causing damage to their bowels by eating offending foods, but this is not the case. As we've said before, bowel damage will not result from eating trigger foods, only symptoms will increase. This is why we can comfortably say that it is your choice to eat trigger foods.

The Low-Caffeine Diet: Who Needs Jumper Cables?

The low-caffeine diet is particularly relevant to people with irritable bowel because caffeine is a stimulant to the muscles in the digestive tract. You know how caffeine stimulates your brain—it wakes you up. It has a similar effect on the digestive tract. Caffeine can cause diarrhea, heartburn, stomach pain, and, in some cases, gas. You don't need to have irritable bowel to have a problem tolerating coffee. However, irritable bowel is particularly susceptible to the effects of caffeine.

Caffeine has been part of our diet for centuries. It is found naturally in plants such as coffee, tea, and cocoa and is added to soft drinks and nonprescription medications. Caffeine behaves like a natural diuretic, which means that it causes fluids to move quickly through the kidneys. Interestingly, this effect may make it more difficult for bran to combine with water to form a soft stool.

The major source of caffeine in our diet is coffee, with colas (dark soft drinks) running a close second. Brewed coffee—the coffee sold in most coffee shops and restaurants and often the coffee of choice at home—contains the most caffeine (see the table on page 104 for the caffeine content of selected beverages). Not surprisingly, decaffeinated coffee is the lowest in caffeine. Even so, decaffeinated coffee can cause just as much stomach acid secretion as regular brew. Therefore, if you experience stomach pain or heartburn as a result of drinking coffee, you may find that even decaf brings no relief. If this is the case, it is best to remove all coffee from your diet.

For most adults, the caffeine in two 6-ounce mugs of coffee per day generally causes no harmful effects. If you can drink this much without experiencing diarrhea, heartburn, and stomach pain, great. But don't drink any more. Many people, though, find that even less coffee causes their irritable bowel symptoms to be worse. If caffeine seems to trigger your symptoms, we advise that you remove coffee from your diet. Giving up or reducing your caffeine intake is a challenge, so we have compiled a list of strategies to help you.

Low-Caffeine Guidelines

Caffeine is a drug. We can become dependent on it. Therefore, giving it up or significantly limiting the caffeine in our diet is easier said than done. However, the benefits of eliminating or significantly decreasing the caffeine in your diet will be well worth the effort, especially if you are prone to diarrhea, heartburn, or stomach pain.

Coffee

1. You might be one of those people who has more success when you give up something all at once. If this is your style, great; your digestive tract will like you. If you go cold turkey, you might experience headaches and tiredness initially, but this disappears in seven to ten days. If you prefer a more gradual approach, see item 2 of this list.

2. You might want to start by trying to stop drinking coffee after a certain hour in the day, such as 3 P.M. Once you have successfully done this, try stopping at noon, and work so that you are consuming only one or two cups of coffee per day. If you are still

experiencing symptoms, we suggest that you remove coffee from your diet. You might need more steps in the plan, depending on how much coffee you drink.

3. Mix your regular coffee with decaffeinated, initially drinking the same number of cups per day. Once you have adjusted to half regular/half decaf, you may gradually work on decreasing both the amount of regular coffee as well as the number of cups of coffee in your diet daily.

4. Mix your coffee with equal amounts of milk while keeping the size of your cup the same. This has the added bonus of getting more milk in your diet. After drinking half coffee/half milk for a while, you can then work on decreasing the number of cups of coffee that you drink daily.

5. Switch to instant coffee, which has half the caffeine content of filter drip. The two are not equal in flavor, but remember that you are trying to give up coffee. After you switch most of your coffee intake to instant, reduce the number of cups you have each day.

6. Replace your coffee with herbal tea. Herbal tea is caffeine free and is much like consuming water. The bonus with herbal tea is that it contributes to your caffeine-free liquid intake. Plus, you still get to enjoy a hot beverage. There are many herbal teas on the market, so you may need to experiment with flavors before you find the ones you like.

Cola

1. Smooth the switch to a noncola soft drink by first choosing decaffeinated colas or light-colored soft drinks. If one of your irritable bowel symptoms is a lot of gas production, switching to a noncola soft drink *will not help* relieve this symptom. You will be better off removing or severely reducing the soft drinks in your diet no matter what the flavor.

2. Replace some of your cola intake with ice water, which is very thirst quenching and counts toward your daily caffeine-free liquid intake. You might even use some juices to satisfy your thirst. This is a very healthy choice. Keep in mind that excessive juice intake (more than three 8-ounce glasses per day) can cause loose bowel movements.

CAFFEINE CONTENT OF SELECTED BEVERAGES

Sources of Caffeine	Caffeine (mg)
Coffee	
Café latte, 8 oz.	50
Cappuccino, 4 oz.	35
Decaf, brewed or instant, 6 oz.	2
Drip, 6 oz.	110
Espresso, 2 oz.	125
Tea	
Black, four-minute brew, 6 oz.	38
Decaf, 6 oz.	2
Green, 4-minute brew, 6 oz.	36
Iced tea, instant, 6 oz.	25
Cola beverage	
Cola or diet cola, 12 oz.	23–31

Source: *Bowes & Church's Food Values of Portions Commonly Used.* 2005. 18th edition. Baltimore, MD: Lippincott Williams & Wilkins.

The Low-Fat Diet: Lose the Fat

The low-fat diet will help reduce symptoms of abdominal pain and diarrhea. But how low does a low-fat diet need to go? The good news here is that you do not need to eat any less fat than is recommended for the general population. The Dietary Guidelines for Americans recommends that fat represent 20 to 35 percent of your daily calorie intake, with most fats coming from healthy sources (see "Oils Group" in chapter 5 for healthy choices). Less than 10 percent of the total intake should come from saturated fat (fat from animal sources such as dairy products, beef, chicken, pork, and eggs, and hydrogenated fats) and trans fat intake should be as low as possible. Your bowels do not recognize the difference between types of fat (saturated versus unsaturated versus trans), but your heart and blood vessels do. Therefore, this low-fat diet is low in total, saturated, and trans fats.

Beyond the amount of fat consumed over a period of days, it is important to limit the amount of fat in a particular meal or snack. Fat is better tolerated when eaten in small amounts throughout the day. Fat is hard to digest, and large amounts can cause the bowel to be irritable.

Low-Fat Guidelines

1. Limit your fat intake from visible fats.
   - Lightly spread margarine or butter (1 teaspoon or less).
   - Choose light margarine.
   - Use jam or jelly rather than margarine or butter.
   - Choose low-fat or fat-free mayonnaise and salad dressings.
   - Choose low-fat or fat-free sour cream.
2. Choose low-fat dairy products.
   - Drink skim or 1 percent milk.
   - Choose fat-reduced yogurt.
   - Choose fat-reduced cheese such as low-fat cheese, which contains less than 20 percent milk fat, or skim milk cheese, which contains less than 7 percent milk fat.
   - Choose frozen yogurt, low-fat ice cream, or frozen ice milk.
3. Choose lean meats and use low-fat cooking methods.
   - Lean cuts of beef—round, sirloin, blade, lean ground, filet, or stew meat.
   - Lean cuts of chicken—skinless chicken breasts and other cuts with skin and fat removed before cooking.
   - Lean cuts of pork—tenderloin, loin chops, and ham with fat removed before eating.
   - Lean cooking methods—barbecuing, baking, broiling, roasting, stewing, steaming, and braising.
4. Choose lower-fat sandwich fillings.
   - Lean fillings—sliced beef, chicken, ham, pastrami, turkey, and low-fat cheese.
   - Use low-fat mayonnaise in egg, tuna, chicken, or salmon salad.
   - Pass on margarine or butter for the bread—choose low-fat mayonnaise or a variety of mustards.
5. Watch out for hidden fats.
   - Make low-fat or reduced-fat muffins, biscuits, pancakes, and waffles rather than buying their higher-fat versions from the

bakery or grocery store. (See the appendix for high-fiber, low-fat recipes.)

- Buy low-fat bakery goods.
- Choose crackers with no more than 5 grams of fat per serving. Even whole wheat crackers can contain hidden fat.
- Avoid crackers made with tropical oils such as coconut, palm, or palm kernel. These are highly saturated and bad for your heart. Avoid crackers that contain trans fat as well.

The greatest source of dietary fat comes from fats that we spread on or add to foods, such as margarine, butter, mayonnaise, salad dressings, and oil. These fats are called *visible fats* because we can see them. We can usually control how much visible fat we consume. For this reason, making changes here can significantly reduce the fat content of your diet.

Another strategy to significantly reduce your fat intake is to choose low-fat dairy products. It is important that we consume dairy products, but we are recognizing that it is equally important to consume those products that are lower in fat. All grocery stores carry low-fat milk, cheese, and yogurt. In fact, the selection has never been better. You will find a variety of spreadable and hard cheeses, yogurt, and frozen yogurts on the shelves. Experiment with a few that you have never tried. We believe that you will find low-fat cheeses and yogurts that you enjoy just as much as the full-fat varieties.

North Americans are known for their fondness for sandwiches: subs, clubs, burgers, heroes, and old standbys of sliced meats and cheese. Cut the fat in your diet by choosing low-fat sandwich fillings and watching the amount of visible fat you put on them.

Finally, as you follow the low-fat diet for irritable bowel, watch out for the hidden fats in foods. Hidden fats are fats that you don't necessarily see; they are present in significant amounts in certain foods such as crackers, muffins, biscuits, and other baked items. Choose low-fat crackers and muffins. (See the appendix for high-fiber, low-fat recipes.)

The Low-Spice Diet: Who Needs Spice in Their Life?

The question of spicy or not spicy foods is common among people with irritable bowel. Everyone tolerates spicy foods differently—irritable bowel or not. However, we have found that those with irritable bowel may not tolerate the following spices:

- Chili powder
- Hot chili peppers
- Garlic
- Hot sauce
- Curry
- Ginger
- Spicy barbecue sauce

You may tolerate these spices in small amounts, but if they are prominent in a dish, you may experience gas, bloating, and diarrhea. We cannot provide exact amounts that you will tolerate. It is up to you to experiment with spices if you are not already certain what types and amounts you can tolerate. If you choose to experiment, we suggest that you start with smaller amounts (see pages 75–77 for testing your tolerance to foods).

Some people mistakenly believe that herbs are difficult to digest. On the contrary, herbs such as basil, oregano, thyme, and rosemary are usually well tolerated if you have irritable bowel. It's usually the other foods in a dish that cause symptoms. For example, lasagna, which can be very high in fat depending on the type and amount of meat and cheese used, can also contain lots of garlic. The high-fat content, garlic, or tomato sauce may cause a person to have abdominal pain, diarrhea, or heartburn. To add flavor to your diet, you may want to experiment with herbs.

The Antireflux Diet: Moving in the Right Direction

You need to be concerned with the antireflux diet only if you have heartburn. Officially, heartburn is not a symptom of irritable bowel, but it is associated with it. Heartburn is the pain you get in your upper chest after acidic stomach contents back up (reflux) into your esophagus.

Normally, stomach contents leave your stomach and enter your small bowel, but with heartburn they travel back into your esophagus. Your stomach and small bowel are designed to handle an acidic environment, but your esophagus is not, so you get that burning sensation when acids make contact with the lining of your esophagus (just as your skin would burn if touched by an acid).

Heartburn is a fairly common problem in North America. It affects an estimated 30 percent or more of all adults—7 percent on a daily basis. Heartburn occurs for a number of reasons, though not all people who have heartburn have irritable bowel. Sometimes stomach contents reflux because of a hiatal hernia, a condition where part of the upper stomach protrudes above the diaphragm. However, many people who have a hiatal hernia do not have symptoms of heartburn. Another possible cause of heartburn is a weak lower esophageal sphincter (LES). This muscle sits at the bottom of the esophagus, where the esophagus meets the stomach. The LES opens when we swallow and closes right after the food and liquid passes into the stomach. If the muscle is weak, though, it does not close effectively, and acidic stomach contents can reflux into the esophagus and cause heartburn.

Antireflux Guidelines

1. Avoid the following foods, which are likely causes of heartburn:
   - Caffeine—particularly coffee, strong tea, and cola beverages
   - Citrus fruits—orange, grapefruit, lemon, and lime
   - Tomatoes—in any form
   - Fatty foods, including fried foods; fatty meats such as bologna, salami, and regular hamburger; and potato chips, peanuts, ice cream, and rich desserts
2. Avoid other trigger foods, including:
   - Alcohol
   - Peppermint
   - Chocolate
   - Spicy foods
3. Wait at least two hours after eating before lying down; a bedtime snack may not be tolerated.
4. Try eating smaller meals; plan to snack midmorning or midafternoon if you get hungry.
5. Drink most fluids between meals.
6. You may need to limit your intake of gas-forming foods such as:

Apples, unpeeled   Broccoli

Beans   Brussels sprouts

Cabbage	Onions
Cantaloupe	Peas, dried
Cauliflower	Raw vegetables, including salads
Corn	Soybeans
Green peppers	Turnips
Honeydew and watermelon	

The goals of the antireflux guidelines are to remove food triggers that cause the LES to weaken and to make some general lifestyle changes that minimize reflux. The first order of dietary treatment is to remove from your diet the notorious trigger foods for heartburn. If you are a coffee lover, you may want to go decaffeinated. However, decaf does trigger acid secretion just like regular coffee, so, it may not provide relief from heartburn. Your best bet then is to remove coffee from your diet (see page 102 for tips) or limit it to one cup per day if you feel that you cannot give it up. That one cup may still cause heartburn, but as with all potential trigger foods, it is your choice to keep it in your diet.

Citrus fruits and their juices are not well tolerated in people who have heartburn. You may want to try other fruit juices such as apple or cranberry, which are sometimes perceived as being less acidic. A number of patients tell us that they cannot drink juice of any kind without getting heartburn. Before removing all juices from your diet, we recommend that you try noncitrus juices that are fortified with vitamin C.

Tomatoes are a major cause of heartburn. Unfortunately, it does not matter in what form you consume them—soup, salad, sandwich, or sauce. The best advice is to avoid tomatoes in all forms.

Fatty foods often trigger heartburn in susceptible people. By fatty foods we mean fried foods such as fried chicken, fried hamburgers, fried steak, fried fish (especially in batter), or french fries. Other fatty foods include salami, pepperoni, regular hamburgers, and bologna; high-fat snacks such as potato chips, tortilla chips, and peanuts; and rich desserts and ice cream. Pasta made with a cream sauce or casseroles made with a cream or cheese sauce may also be high in fat and cause heartburn.

Besides the main heartburn triggers, a few foods are what we call secondary triggers of heartburn: alcohol, peppermint, chocolate, and spicy foods. These substances may not trigger heartburn in all people if consumed in small amounts. After six weeks, you may want to check your tolerance to these substances (see pages 75–77 for more information on testing your tolerance to foods).

Your chance of heartburn can also be lowered if you wait at least two hours after eating before you lie down. Stomach contents are more likely to reflux into your esophagus when you lie down. When people wake up with heartburn in the middle of the night, it's usually because they ate an evening snack. If you are accustomed to a bedtime snack, you will need to eat it two or more hours earlier, and make it a light snack, such as a small bowl of cereal or a slice of toast. You may even find that you can't eat an evening snack at all without waking up with heartburn. In this case, it is best to avoid snacking in the evening. Another strategy for reducing heartburn and acid reflux at night is to sleep with the head of the bed elevated about 6 inches.

Sometimes people feel better and have less heartburn if they eat small meals and snack if they get hungry. You are more likely to reflux after a large meal because an overdistended stomach puts pressure on the food to move upward. Drinking a lot of fluid (more than two 8-ounce glasses) with meals may cause reflux. Try to keep your liquid intake with meals or snacks equal to or less than this amount.

Finally, some gassy foods may reflux into your esophagus, though this is not common. In the interest of thoroughness, we have included this possibility. Should you find that a variety of gassy vegetables and fruits cause you to have heartburn, see pages 95–101 for guidelines about low gassy foods and advice on meeting your nutritional requirements.

More Diet Adjustments

There are a few more diet adjustments you may want to know about if you are intolerant of alcohol or lactose.

Alcohol: More Than an Appetite Stimulant

We are often asked about the effects of alcohol on irritable bowel. As mentioned earlier, alcohol is a stimulant to your digestive tract. It gets your digestive juices going and enhances your appetite (this is the function of the before-dinner drink called the aperitif). For people with irritable bowel, alcohol may cause symptoms such as heartburn, stomach pain, and/or diarrhea.

We usually advise people to drink alcohol in moderation to minimize its effects. Moderate alcohol consumption equals no more than one drink per day for women and no more than two drinks per day for men. One drink is equivalent to 5 ounces of wine, 12 ounces of beer, or 1½ ounces of 80-proof spirits. For people who cannot drink even a small amount of alcohol without increasing their irritable bowel symptoms, it's best to avoid all alcoholic beverages to feel well.

We have stated before that it is your choice whether you consume potentially offending foods and beverages, but you need to prepare yourself for the consequences of increased symptoms. Alcohol is unique in that it is a harmful substance if consumed in excess. In addition, some people should not drink alcoholic beverages for specific health reasons such as liver or pancreatic disease or while taking certain medications. If you do not already know whether it is okay for you to drink alcohol, check with your doctor.

Lactose: The Suspected Sugar

Another food item that is often the reason for diet adjustments is lactose. Some people cannot tolerate this natural milk sugar. Symptoms of lactose intolerance are gas, bloating, and, in 50 percent of cases, diarrhea—anywhere from fifteen minutes to two hours after lactose is consumed.

Milk sugar is normally broken down into smaller sugars and absorbed in the small bowel. People who are lactose intolerant do not break all the milk sugar down, so when lactose gets to the large bowel, bacteria digest it and produce gases in the process. This causes people to feel gassy and bloated. Diarrhea may also occur because many little sugar molecules that should not be in the large bowel attract water to the bowel, and hence watery stools result.

Lactose intolerance is a separate condition from irritable bowel. However, as you can see, it may have similar symptoms—namely gas, bloating, and diarrhea. In fact, irritable bowel symptoms frequently are mistaken for lactose intolerance. This may lead to the unnecessary avoidance of milk products and potential nutrient deficiencies. We see many people in our clinic who needlessly avoid milk products. It is important to sort out whether you are lactose intolerant or have irritable bowel, or both.

Lactose intolerance is more prevalent in certain populations and is more likely to be a causal factor in digestive symptoms among Asian and African adults, who have an estimated prevalence rate of 90 percent.

Your local hospital or health clinic can conduct several tests to diagnose lactose intolerance. The two most common are the hydrogen breath test and the lactose tolerance test. Most often, lactose intolerance is diagnosed by removing lactose from the diet and assessing whether symptoms go away. This may not be helpful, though, since lactose intolerance symptoms can be similar to those of irritable bowel. Still, if you are lactose intolerant, removing lactose from your diet should significantly reduce your gas, bloating, and diarrhea, even if they do not go away entirely.

Generally, people are not 100 percent lactose intolerant. Most people with lactose intolerance can handle small amounts of lactose, such as milk in tea or coffee, the lactose in hard cheese, the milk solids in margarine, and the milk in a piece of cake or a muffin. Many people tolerate a small amount of milk (½ cup) for cereal and the milk solids present in yogurt.

Determining If You Are Lactose Intolerant

If you have gas, bloating, and diarrhea or loose (watery) stools, you can determine whether you are lactose intolerant by having a test as noted earlier or you can remove lactose from your diet for a two- to three-week trial (see also pages 75–77).

If you remove lactose-containing foods from your diet, target milk, cream, puddings, yogurt, frozen yogurt, ice cream, and all types of cheese. If you feel you cannot do without milk in your tea or coffee, use low-lactose milk (you can buy this in your local grocery store). Watch to see if your symptoms diminish or go away. If you do not feel any different, lactose intolerance is not the problem, and you can feel free to enjoy a variety of milk products.

If after removing lactose-containing foods from your diet you feel like you have less bloating, gas, and diarrhea, you may be lactose intolerant. The next step is to determine how lactose intolerant you are. Can you put milk in tea or coffee? Can you have a small amount of milk on your cereal? Can you eat yogurt or enjoy hard cheese? The best way to test this is to try a lactose-containing item in small amounts, such as 1 to 2 ounces of hard cheese, ½ cup of yogurt, or ½ cup of milk with cereal. You may well find that you can enjoy lactose-containing foods only in small amounts.

If you are lactose intolerant, it would be wise to choose a low-lactose milk to ensure that you meet your requirement for calcium. Low-lactose milk should be available at your local grocery store. You can also buy a lactase enzyme at your pharmacy, which breaks down the lactose.

Lactose intolerance and milk allergy are not the same thing. People who are allergic to milk have an allergic reaction (a specific chemical response) to the proteins in milk. Milk allergy in adults is very rare. In the case of milk allergy, all milk products need to be avoided and a calcium supplement is necessary.

Meeting Your Calcium Needs

We find that the majority of women who come to our clinic do not consume enough calcium. Actually, this isn't so unusual when you consider that for many North Americans calcium content of the diet is less than recommended. This is particularly disconcerning because a poor calcium intake over time results in weak bones that are prone to fracture. Compounding this for women is the hormonal change of decreased estrogen at menopause, which causes accelerated loss of calcium from the bone.

A diet deficient in calcium is one of the risk factors for osteoporosis, a condition where your bones become porous and fragile and may fracture or break easily. One in four women will develop osteoporosis. Increasing calcium just at menopause has a limited effect on preventing osteoporosis, so it's best if you seek calcium early in life, especially as a teenager and young adult.

Milk, cheese, and yogurt are the best sources of calcium. If you do not consume adequate dairy products, it will be difficult to get the calcium your body needs. You may require a calcium supplement. An expert panel of nutrition scientists from Canada and the United States studied nutrients for bone health and recommend 1,000 milligrams of calcium daily for people between the ages of nineteen and fifty and 1,200 to 1,500 milligrams for those age fifty-one and older. Milk also contains vitamin D. The recommended amount of vitamin D is 200 international units (IU) per day until age fifty, 400 IU for people between the ages of fifty-one and seventy, and 600 IU for those over the age of seventy.

8

What Is Stress, and Does It Affect Irritable Bowel?

Irritable bowel is a complex and potentially confusing condition. Once symptoms develop, you will likely seek help from a physician. This is the usual entry point into the diagnosis, assessment, and control of irritable bowel symptoms for most people. We support this, since it is important to make sure that there is nothing medically wrong with your bowel (a bowel disease) before you try learning to live with irritable bowel (a condition in which your bowel is normal but easily irritated).

So the first message you get is that irritable bowel is a medical problem (true). Next, the issue of how food affects your irritable bowel gets raised. So the second message you get is that irritable bowel is a food-related problem (also true). Once food issues are considered, the possible role of stress is introduced. So the third message you get is that irritable bowel is a stress-related problem (again true). It is never immediately clear which of these factors—medical, food-related or stress-related, or their combination—is disrupting the normal functioning of your gut. The point here is twofold. First, it can be confusing for people to figure out which approach is best for them, and second, stress can get downplayed for some people (it usually comes third in line). In this chapter, we will focus on the issue of stress and its potential relationship to irritable bowel.

"Stress" is a word that is familiar to us all. In fact, we use the word *stress* so often that it is not clear whether stress is a good thing or a bad thing. We hear people say that they are constantly stressed out, that the world is becoming more and more stressful, and that stress is a problem for most of us. But is stress always bad? The answer is no. When does manageable stress ("I'm doing okay"), or even a positive stress, which might be experienced as an exciting challenge ("I can't wait to do that again"), become interfering distress ("I can't take it anymore")?

Although *stress* is an overused word, we should not throw out the baby with the bathwater. In this chapter, we will teach you about stress: how to define it, how to assess your own stress level, and, most importantly, how to reduce stress. Let us start with some common questions.

What Does Stress Mean?

At its basic level, stress refers to the body's reaction to a challenge or threat. Anything that challenges the body (and remember, the mind is part of the body) is stressful. We categorize stress by the part of the body that is being challenged. Running up a flight of stairs stresses the muscles and the heart (a physical stress); confronting a critical boss for a raise stresses you mentally (an emotional or cognitive stress). Even though the stress might start out as physical (or mental), however, one system affects the other. For example, if, when driving home tonight you encounter a traffic accident as it happens, you might rush out of your car and lend help, without much thought (your body will be stressed). Once you get home, however, you might begin to feel distressed (mental stress). Your initial reaction is physical; after you've had a chance to think about it the stress becomes mental. Psychological stress takes many forms, and it has been repeatedly shown in research studies that stress can affect the functioning of the gut.

How Does Stress Affect the Gut?

Stress affects the functioning of the digestive tract in several ways (see chapter 3 for general information about how the gut works). When stressed, the body reacts automatically by engaging the so-called fight-or-flight response. This response is the body's way of getting ready to take action. Your body is like a fire department. When a fire alarm goes off, the fire department responds as quickly as possible. The fire department treats all alarms as serious, regardless of whether the alarm is false or real. The stress response is one of the body's alarm systems. When stress is perceived, the body prepares for action whether there is a need for action (for example, you run to get away from an attacking dog that wanders into your backyard while you are barbecuing) or not (for example, the way you feel when you think someone has insulted you but he or she clarifies that he or she was actually talking about someone else—you still feel the insult).

To prepare you for action, several things happen in your body. Your muscles tighten, your heart rate and breathing speed up, and stress hormones (for example, adrenaline) are released. Each of these normal reactions can affect your gut. Muscle tension can alter the normal rhythms of your bowel, leading to altered bowel habits, such as constipation and diarrhea, or to heartburn. One way to think about your gut is to imagine an orchestra. When all the instruments are working properly and playing together (the horns come in when they are supposed to, the drum stops at the right moment), beautiful music results. If, however, the timing is thrown off (the horns come in when the drums are supposed to, not all the violins play at the same time), you have nothing but painful, irritating noise. This is how the gut works as well. That is why you can have no disease (all the instruments are in good working order) but very intense symptoms that interfere with your ability to function and cope (the orchestra makes nothing but painful noise).

Since stress has such a strong effect on the body, many people with irritable bowel need to learn to manage and reduce stress. This is true both for positive stresses (the challenge of a new job or anxiously awaiting your wedding day) and negative stresses (losing your job or worrying about finances). Managing stress differs depending on the type and causes of stress. In this chapter, we will talk about two types of stress. First, there are the stresses that interfere with normal bowel functioning and directly result in bowel symptoms (direct stress effect). Stress will directly upset the gut for some people. Also, your pattern of coping with stress can disrupt normal gut functioning if you cope by overeating or drinking excess coffee or alcohol, or if your sleep is interrupted. Second, there are the stresses that result from having bowel symptoms (indirect stress effects). The best example of this type of stress is the fear of incontinence that is common among those with diarrhea-prone irritable bowel. If you are one of these people, you may find yourself orienting to all the restrooms in the areas that you travel. Being in a new place can be stressful simply because you do not know where there is a restroom.

Besides these types of stresses, we will also concern ourselves with people who are prone to stress. Some people easily become worried and preoccupied about their health even when there is nothing to worry about. I'm sure you know someone who could be described, or who describes him- or herself, as a worrywart. Irritable bowel symptoms are a problem for these people, but only part of the problem, as they worry about other body systems besides the gut (these individuals are called *somatizers*). Also, there are some people who have psychological problems apart from irritable bowel (these people are identified as having psychopathology). The issues faced by those who tend to be somatizers or who have psychopathology are covered in chapter 12.

Assessing Stress

Before we look at the stresses that produce irritable bowel symptoms and the stress caused by irritable bowel symptoms, let's talk about how you can evaluate your own stress level. It is important to accept that stress is subjective. Only you can tell if you are stressed and how stressed you are. Other people might have something valuable to say about how they perceive your level of stress, and it is often useful to consider others' opinions. But in the end it comes down to you judging your own stress level. This is an important point, because other people use their own experiences as a basis to judge others. If someone told you that you were stressed out, it could be true. But then again, it might mean that he or she would feel stressed if he or she were in your situation. Consider bungee jumping. Some people would consider this a terrifying experience and think you would have to be out of your mind to do it. Yet others find it exciting and fun and pay to do it. Who is right? No one; it depends on your point of view.

Take a moment to ask yourself: "How stressed do I feel?" You might have a different answer depending on whether you are talking about this very moment, the past month, or the past year. A good time frame to consider is two months. On page 120 you will find a stress test. You should fill this test out to get an idea of your overall stress level and of some of the stress symptoms that bother you. If there are some symptoms of stress that you don't see listed, don't worry; just make a note of those symptoms. You'll notice that irritable bowel symptoms are not included in this test; we assume that you have these symptoms because you are reading this book. We recommend that you take your time with this part of the workbook. The more thought you put into filling in the tables and charts, the more clearly you will see how stress affects your life.

You will note that, in the end, you assigned yourself to a category of low, moderate, or high stress. This is because only you can determine how much stress is a problem for you. By counting the number of stress symptoms you have, you will be able to determine how much your body responds to stress. Looking at your ratings, you can also judge your overall level of happiness or quality of life. A basic rule would be the more stress symptoms you have, and the more they affect your quality of life, the more helpful stress management will be.

We also need to make you aware that some people with irritable bowel don't experience a lot of stress that they can identify. As you read in chapter 1, your gut may be an early warning system for you. That is, it may be that irritable bowel symptoms are the first indication that you are under stress. If this is true for you, the stress test might not tell you all that much. You will likely learn more from keeping a diary of your symptoms and studying the factors that surround you when and to what extent you have symptoms.

Let's get back to assessing stress in your life. Make a list of the specific things that you consider to be the main stresses in your life, especially the things that you find upsetting. Use the following chart to write down your stresses. Beside each stressful thing, rate how upsetting it is, assigning a number from 1 (not at all upsetting) to 10 (extremely upsetting).

The Stress Test

1   Answer the following questions true or false based on how you have been feeling over the past two months:

> Life is exciting.
>
> I wake up feeling refreshed.
>
> I am calm and relaxed.
>
> I feel in control of my life.

If you answered false to any of the above questions, this chapter is for you. If you answered false to most of the questions, read on carefully.

2.   Rate the following:

> Over the past two months, how happy and content have you been (circle the number):

1	2	3	4	5
Not at all happy		Somewhat happy		Extremely happy

> Over the past two months, how stressed have you felt?

1	2	3	4	5
Not at all stressed		Somewhat stressed		Extremely stressed

3.   Check which of the following stress symptoms you experience. Check only those symptoms that bother you or interfere with your quality of life:

	Yes	No
Feel tense all the time	☐	☐
Can't relax	☐	☐
Disturbed sleep	☐	☐
Worry too much	☐	☐
Can't slow down	☐	☐
Always feel I'm behind	☐	☐
Bothered by constant fatigue	☐	☐

Your responses to these questions should tell you how stressed you are. Remember, stress is subjective.

4.   Put yourself in one of the following three categories. Remember that stress is subjective, and we are asking you for an overall judgment.

Low stress ☐   Moderate stress ☐   High stress ☐

Stress	How Upsetting 1 (not upsetting)– 10 (very upsetting)	Acute or Chronic
1. _____	_____	_____
2. _____	_____	_____
3. _____	_____	_____
4. _____	_____	_____
5. _____	_____	_____
6. _____	_____	_____

Now, for each stress that you wrote down in the chart, ask yourself whether the stressful event is time limited (for example, an upcoming performance review by your boss) or whether the stress has no foreseeable end (for example, an unemployed federal civil servant looking for another job). We call time-limited stressors *acute* stressors, and ones that have no clear end *chronic* stressors. Put an A beside the acute stresses and a C beside the chronic stresses. Chronic stress is more difficult to deal with and often has a greater impact on the body, because the body can never get away from it (even if you can temporarily shut it out of your mind). So if you have a lot of stresses that you rate as chronic, it is likely that stress management will be helpful for you.

Next, ask yourself if there is anything that you can do to alter the stress. For example, if a coworker is insensitive to your needs, you could speak to him or her using assertiveness techniques. An example of a stress that can't be altered is the stress associated with the death of a loved one. If there is something you can do, then it is a *controllable* stress. If there is nothing you can do, it is an *uncontrollable* stress. Uncontrollable stressors are more difficult to deal with than controllable ones. In your list, if you have many uncontrollable stresses that cause moderate, or more, upset, read the next chapter on how to reduce the impact of stress on your body.

If you consider yourself to be stressed, and it has lasted a month or more, ask yourself: "What do I do to cope with stress?" Does it work? In the following chart make a list of the things you do to cope and mark whether they are positive (P) or negative (N), and then rate if they work for you. Do this now.

What you do to cope with stress: **P or N?**

1. _____

   _____   _____

2. _____

   _____   _____

3. _____

   _____

4. _____

   _____

5. _____

   _____

How well do these strategies work?

1	2	3	4	5
Not at all		Somewhat well		Extremely well

What coping strategies would you like to do more of, and what less of?

More   **Less**

_____   _____

_____   _____

_____   _____

_____   _____

_____   _____

Note that some coping strategies can be negative and some positive. Positive coping strategies include sitting down and analyzing a problem, seeking support from others, or exercising. These strategies are positive because they help you and cause no harm. Negative coping strategies may include things like drinking excessive amounts of coffee or alcohol, smoking, or eating to excess. These are negative coping strategies because even though they help you cope, they cause problems themselves. Mark whether your coping strategies are positive or negative by placing a P or an N beside the coping strategy. You might need to ask a friend what he or she thinks, because sometimes we deny unhealthy behavior ("I just drink to relax, I can stop anytime").

Finally, in assessing your stress level, you should be aware of the distinction between *life events stress* and *daily hassles*. Life events stresses are those major events that happen in life that almost anyone would find stressful, such as losing a job; the death of a spouse, a relative, or a close friend; getting married; and moving to a new city. Most of these stresses fall into several categories: finances, relationships, health, and social functioning. These events tend to be relatively easy to identify. Apart from these major events, a very common source of stress is from daily hassles. These are the small things that we often ignore but that can build up and have an accumulated negative effect on our emotions and health. Getting stuck in traffic and being late for an important appointment, being treated rudely by a store clerk, or spilling coffee on your new clothes are all examples of small things that can get under our skin and cause stress. Since these events are minor, we (and others) tend to overlook them. For instance, we tend not to talk to others about these types of events (that is, seek social support) because others are often unsympathetic due to the minor nature of the incidents ("what are you complaining about, we all go though that"). These are the types of events, however, that can build up and add to our stress.

We recognize that this has been a lot of work so far. But you will find that it pays off if you are able to identify your stresses, how they affect you, and how you cope with them.

Self-Monitoring

There is one final point that needs to be raised before we look at coping with stress in more detail. If you are going to be successful in managing stress, you will need to be able to keep track of what is happening regarding the stresses. We call this *self-monitoring*. Most people don't pay close attention to the fine details of their lives. For instance, what did you eat for lunch last Wednesday? Unless you eat the same lunch most days you probably don't remember. There are just too many other things to attend to in a day. Consequently, we don't pay close enough attention and cannot recall small details of our day-to-day activities. Yet, to learn how to change behavior, and to manage stress, you must identify patterns that are called *stress-symptoms associations*. The best way to do this with irritable bowel is to keep a stress diary. A copy of such a diary can be found on pages 126 and 127. Complete this diary for a one-week interval. While this sounds like a lot, you will find that it will be worth the trouble because you will have a much better sense of the role that stress plays. A big part of reducing stress is awareness. If you don't know what the problem is, then solving it is pretty tough. With a clear idea of the problem, solutions are much easier to achieve. You don't have to fill in the diary as things happen, unless that is what you prefer. Most people find that they can fill it in at the end of the day.

Each day, record the intensity of your irritable bowel symptoms, your overall stress level, and the stresses of the day and how they affected you in terms of irritable bowel symptoms. You will also want to record your feelings, your worries, and how you coped with stress. After you complete one week of this diary, you can analyze it to look for connections between stress and symptoms, identify the specific stresses that bother you, and determine your coping techniques. We don't recommend that you try to keep a detailed record for more than one week because most people find it difficult to continue keeping such a record for much longer. Also, we don't recommend that you try to analyze your record until after you've kept it for a week. Stress patterns are often subtle and need to be studied over time.

You might need more space than is provided in this diary. If so, copy it onto a blank piece of paper or make a photocopy. Good luck!

Final Thoughts on Stress

This chapter will help you determine the extent to which you lead a stressful life and if these stresses are a cause of your irritable bowel. It may be the case that stress does not play a major role in the onset of your symptoms. This might be true if your irritable bowel symptoms are primarily caused by foods that you eat. It may still be the case that stress is an important issue to manage to get control of irritable bowel. In chapter 2, you kept a record of your irritable bowel symptoms. By examining when your symptoms happened, you may be able to identify stressful situations. For many people, it is the irritable bowel symptoms that are the first indication of a stressful situation. Also, you may find that the irritable bowel symptoms are a main source of stress for you. This is one of the reasons that irritable bowel is such a challenging condition to manage. The symptoms can be the source of the stress that causes more symptoms. It's like being caught in a vicious cycle: irritable bowel leads to stress, which leads to more irritable bowel, which leads to more stress, which leads to more irritable bowel, and on and on.

There is one final point we would like to make. You will notice that in chapter 6 you are also asked to keep a diary of your eating and irritable bowel symptoms. When you start out with this book, you may want to do one of these diaries but not both. You can start with a food diary or a stress diary. Trying to do both at the same time when you are first learning from this book might be confusing and overwhelming. This is because it takes a lot of effort to keep a diary that will be useful. Also, you may find that the stress and the food diaries overlap. This is true for many reasons. One reason is that if you eat something that causes irritable bowel symptoms, this can be stressful in itself. Also, stress and eating are closely related. We eat not so much for nutrition as we do for comfort or as part of our social world. Many people would describe themselves as emotional eaters, referring to the fact that they will eat when under stress. The food choices that people make when they are under stress are often unhealthy choices. When stressed, you are much more likely to eat chocolate or cookies than you are broccoli or cauliflower. Whichever diary you work on first (stress or food), you will learn how that factor affects your irritable bowel. When you then work on the second diary, you will see how the second factor (food or stress) affects your irritable bowel and how food and stress are connected.

STRESS DIARY

Complete this diary daily for one week. Choose a convenient time each day when you can spend a few minutes to reflect on the day and identify the extent and source of your stress.

	Situation	Severity of Symptoms (1 = minimal/negligible; 10 = extreme severity)	Stress	Stress Level (1 = no stress; 10 = extreme stress)	Coping
Monday					
Tuesday					
Wednesday					

	Situation	Severity of Symptoms (1 = minimal/negligible; 10 = extreme severity)	Stress	Stress Level (1 = no stress; 10 = extreme stress)	Coping
Thursday					
Friday					
Saturday					
Sunday					

9

Stress Management

For many of you, stress management will be essential to helping you successfully cope with irritable bowel. In this chapter, you will learn specific methods for coping with stress. For these methods to be effective, you will need to practice them. The basic principle of coping skills is practice, practice, practice. The biggest reason why stress management methods do not help some people is that these people don't always realize it takes time for the methods to become effective. Think of stress reduction skills as you would about driving skills. You wouldn't get your beginner's permit on Wednesday, go out for your first driving lesson on Thursday, and expect to take and pass your driver's exam on Friday! You need repeated practice to build skill and confidence. It is the same with stress management methods. Also, you wouldn't go onto the highway in rush hour for your first driving lesson. You would go to parking lot at a time when it isn't busy. In the same way, it is best to learn and practice stress management methods when you are calm. Don't expect them to work in stressful situations until you have become confident in your ability to use the methods. Keep in mind that if at first you don't succeed, try, try again.

We will now examine three main stress management strategies: calming your body, calming your mind, and reducing the stress. Because irritable bowel is a condition that involves increased sensitivity of the gut as well as increased body arousal, learning to calm your body is the first step to normalizing the functioning of your gut.

Calming Your Body

As explained in chapters 1 and 2, irritable bowel involves a disruption in the normal rhythms of the gut. Chapter 8 described how stress factors make this worse by further disrupting your gut. As a result, calming your body is critical for helping the gut resume its normal, healthy rhythms (that is, for helping to reduce symptoms). In our experience, it is essential for people with irritable bowel to learn how to keep their bodies calm. Even if you are successful in eliminating the cause of your stress, your body might not automatically return to a state of calm. It is common for people to be unaware of how tense they are. Think about when you start your summer vacation. After a day or so, once you've begun to feel relaxed, you realize how stressed you felt before the vacation. You must learn to reduce your body's level of stress. If you are successful, you can expect reduced pain, discomfort, and distress, and more normal bowel function (that is, less diarrhea/constipation, bloating, and gas). Two strategies are important to calm your body: deep breathing and deep muscle relaxation.

Deep Breathing

Stop reading for a moment and take a deep breath. Now, take another breath.

Pay attention to the parts of your body that move as you breathe. Put your hand on your chest and take another deep breath. Did your hand move as you breathed in? Take another breath and observe whether your chest moves up as you breathe in. If your hand on your chest moved up when you breathed in, you are breathing *wrong*. If you paused, even slightly, between breathing in and out, you are breathing *wrong*.

In our clinical work, when we ask our patients to do this exercise, 99 percent of them breathe incorrectly. Breathing by using your chest muscles does not allow you to take a deep breath. Chest breathing is called *shallow breathing.* Some people can even hyperventilate by chest breathing, which can cause a panic attack. We learn to breathe with our chest muscles because it is easy to control these muscles, and shallow breathing makes it easier to talk and breathe at the same time.

Learning deep breathing methods is very effective in relaxing the body for a number of reasons. First, it slows down the rate of breathing; this has a very calming effect. Second, deep breathing makes better use of your lung capacity; you get more air in each breath. Because there is more air in the lungs, your heart rate slows down (it doesn't have to move the blood as quickly) and your blood pressure lowers (the blood doesn't have to be forced through your body as hard). So there are both psychological and physical benefits from deep breathing. To breathe deeply, you need to use your stomach muscles, not your chest muscles.

Sit up straight, put both feet on the floor in front of you, and put one hand on your chest and the other hand on your stomach. Now, push in with your lower hand and resist this push—feel those muscles? These are the muscles that you use to breathe deeply.

Deep breathing involves two steps:

1. Breathe *in* through your nose, pushing your stomach *out.*
2. Breathe *out* through your mouth, pulling your stomach *in.*

Notice that your chest muscles are not used in deep breathing. Now take a few minutes, review these instructions, and practice deep breathing. By keeping one hand on your chest and one on your stomach you can guide yourself through the exercise.

Keep your chest hand still and allow your stomach hand to move in and out.

You might also want to practice deep breathing by lying flat on your back, placing a small book (a thin paperback is ideal) on your lower stomach (just below your belly button) and making the book go up when you breathe in and down when you breathe out.

Most people find that when they first try to follow these deep breathing exercises they feel worse, not better. This is because your normal breathing pattern is being disrupted. The solution to this is to practice. You should not expect this (or any other methods listed in this book) to work immediately. Remember, you shouldn't try to learn deep breathing when you are highly stressed. First learn it when you are calm. Once you are skilled at it, you can use it to reduce stress.

Deep breathing, once learned, can be an extremely effective method for calming you. This is because it is simple, and once learned, can be implemented virtually anywhere, anytime. More important, slowing down your breathing rate by using this method reduces your heart rate and blood pressure, and this directly calms you. Once you have become comfortable with this method, you should practice it daily. Since it is so simple and quick, you should be able to use it whenever you're feeling stressed. As a way of helping you learn how to use this method, you could try using it the next time you're driving. Whenever you hit a red light, take two or three deep breaths. You'll see that it will keep you calm.

Deep Muscle Relaxation

The second method you need to learn to reduce irritable bowel symptoms is deep muscle relaxation. This method is very effective because it directly reduces muscle tension. Increased muscle tension can disturb the functioning of the gut because the bowel is like a big muscle in the shape of a tube. There are many ways to relax, and many people find their own way. Some people take long baths, others go for a stroll in the woods, others practice tai chi, and so on. Usually, however, these methods of relaxation are difficult to incorporate into our busy lives, and we do them only on occasion. Also, many of these methods might result in mental relaxation but not physical relaxation. Deep muscle relaxation can relax the body directly by focusing on the muscles themselves. At first, this method takes fifteen to twenty minutes to complete. Once learned, however, you can accomplish relaxation in a much shorter time.

As with deep breathing, you need to become skilled in muscle relaxation before you can expect it to work. In our clinical practice, we tell people that they should practice relaxation daily for ten to fourteen days when they are calm before they can expect it to work. Giving up too early is a major problem. Think of these coping skills like investing in a retirement plan: you don't get the returns until down the road, but when they come in they are worth the wait.

Deep muscle relaxation is such an effective method for managing irritable bowel because of its direct effect on muscle tension. The bowel is easily affected by tension. After all, the bowel is like one big muscle, but one that moves in a special way. Fecal material is moved through the bowel by peristaltic movements. If you've ever had to get a drawstring out of a waistband when it has slipped inside the front opening (as with a pair of sweatpants), you know about these kinds of contractions. This is also how a snake eats its food. Muscle tension can throw off the timing of this very complicated muscle movement. Tension and stress can also throw off the timing of secretions throughout the stomach and the bowel, which contributes further to symptoms. Physically relaxing these muscles can allow the normal rhythms of the bowel to resume.

Learning how to relax involves learning how to detect when your muscles are tense.

Take your left hand, make a fist, and squeeze slightly, not hard. Pay attention to the sensations associated with this tension. Now let go of the tension gradually. Now do this again, only don't squeeze as hard as the first time, and let go of the tension much more slowly.

Learning to identify when muscles are tense and letting go of the tension is the method of relaxation. You can learn to identify tension by learning to scan your body. Let's practice this first.

Take a slow deep breath, clear your mind, and focus your attention on your body.

The first time you read this it will be difficult because you will need to divide your attention between reading and following the instructions. After you've read this a few times, you will get the hang of it and be able to do it without reading. Once you are familiar with these instructions, scan your body with your eyes closed.

Your attention is like the beacon of a spotlight, and you can control its direction. Focus your attention on the sensations in the bottom of your feet (hold this for five seconds). Now focus your attention on the sensations in your neck (hold this for five seconds). Now focus your sensations on your fingers (hold this for five seconds).

Notice that as you move your attention from one part of your body to another the sensations in each part of your body become stronger and easier to identify. Learning to scan your body in this way will help you identify areas of tension, areas that you can pay special attention to as you learn deep muscle relaxation.

Starting at your head, scan your body to identify areas of tension. We don't want you to add tension, just become aware of the tension that is already there. Focus on your head . . . neck . . . shoulders . . . arms . . . chest . . . stomach . . . back . . . buttocks . . . legs . . . and feet. Do you feel tightness, tension, or pain in any of these areas?

Many people report that certain body parts are associated with tension for them. The most common are the jaw, the top of head, the shoulders, and the back.

The best way to understand how to relax is to learn how to let go of tension in specific muscle groups. To do this, you should first add a small amount of tension to that muscle group. By adding this tension voluntarily, you can voluntarily let go of that tension. If you add a small amount of tension for a short period (five to ten seconds) and then let go of that tension very gradually over a longer period (thirty to forty-five seconds), you will reduce the level of tension in that muscle group to a level lower than where it was when you started. *That's the trick to deep muscle relaxation!*

Putting It All Together

Find a comfortable place, away from noise and distractions (turn off the television or radio), where you can lie flat, so you don't have to hold up any part of your body, such as your head or arms. A bed or recliner is perfect for this. Loosen any tight-fitting clothing and get comfortable. You should read these instructions a couple of times to become familiar with them and then put this book down to try the procedure.

To achieve a relaxed state, you need to work through a series of muscle groups. Each muscle group should be put through the tense-relax cycle twice before you move on to the next muscle group. The following muscle groups are involved:

- Hands and forearms (both left and right)
- Shoulder muscles
- Neck muscles

- Forehead muscles
- Jaw muscles
- Stomach muscles
- Back muscles
- Buttocks
- Thigh/hamstring muscles
- Feet/calf muscles

First, tense your hands and forearms (a small amount) and study the tension (five to ten seconds maximum). Now relax and focus on gradually easing the tension. Keep in mind the image of a flower and the petals of the flower opening in the morning sun; they don't pop open suddenly, but gradually and smoothly. This is how you should relax your muscles.

Repeat this procedure for each of the listed muscle groups. It should take you about twenty to twenty-five minutes to go through all of them. It is not important that you feel extremely relaxed after doing this, especially the first few times. What is critical is that you can feel some degree of relaxation (that is, you know you are more relaxed at the end than when you started). If you can achieve this, then deep relaxation will come with practice.

To learn how to relax you need to be aware of the following:

1. *When muscles are tense.* To learn this, practice scanning your body, that is, focusing your attention inward at specific muscle groups.
2. *Adding a small amount of tension.* It is critical that you do not tense too hard, but just enough to notice an increase.
3. *Letting go of the tension.* This is where the method pays off. Learning to slowly let go of tension brings immediate relief and calmness. Be sure to let go slowly and smoothly. The following are some guidelines for tensing your muscles:

Muscle Group:	Tense By:
Hands and forearms	Make a fist and squeeze
Shoulders	Lift your shoulders up and hold
Neck	Push your head back into the chair or bed

Forehead	Raise your eyebrows
Jaw	Put your jaws together
Stomach	Make you stomach hard (as if you were going to be punched)
Back	Push your shoulder blades back
Buttocks	Tighten your bum
Thighs and hamstrings	Tighten your upper legs
Feet and calves	Point your toes toward your head or away from your body

Imagery

Before moving on, we should also talk about using your imagination to relax. This form of relaxation involves distraction. Some people have very active imaginations and can use them to calm themselves. To do this, take three to five minutes and find a comfortable place where you won't be disturbed. Read the following instructions several times, until you become familiar with them, and then practice the method.

Close your eyes and create a picture in your mind's eye. Imagine a calm, relaxing scene, such as lying on a sandy Caribbean beach, with the sun beating down on your skin and a warm breeze in your hair. Use all your senses to create this image: see the white sand, with the sun glittering off each tiny grain; see the green-blue of the ocean; hear the wind in the palm trees and the far-off call of seabirds; smell the salt air; feel the heat of the sun and the grains of sand under your feet; taste the salt on your tongue from the sea breeze.

By involving all your senses, you will become more involved in the image, and it will be more distracting to you. Most people find that an image will stay clearly in their mind for twenty to thirty seconds before breaking up. This is normal. When it happens, simply re-create the image by asking yourself the same questions (what do I hear, see, feel, smell, and taste?).

Imagery can be a useful strategy because your imagination is boundless. Be creative and have *fun*. The types of images that people most often find useful are relaxing images (a beach), exciting images (skiing on a sunny day), or detailed images (imagining all the colors in a rainbow).

Calming Your Mind

By using the previous methods, you can calm your body, which will help reduce irritable bowel symptoms. But often that is not enough. This is because a great deal of stress is produced by our tendency to worry or catastrophize (think in terms of worst-case, or catastrophic, scenarios). It has been demonstrated in several clinical studies that our thinking patterns have a strong influence over our emotions, behavior, and bowel symptoms. By monitoring our stress reactions and looking for thoughts associated with symptoms, or with feelings of stress, we can identify patterns of thinking that contribute to and worsen irritable bowel symptoms. Once we have proven to ourselves that our thinking patterns relate to our symptoms, we can work to alter our thinking style. This is not simply the power of positive thinking; it is a method of analyzing our thoughts and thinking them through from a different perspective. Three steps are involved: self-monitoring, self-analysis, and changing your thoughts (psychologists call this cognitive restructuring).

Self-Monitoring

As with so many other aspects of managing irritable bowel, you need to study your own situation to identify how your symptoms are produced and controlled. Keeping a record of irritable bowel episodes and stressful events, with an eye toward identifying thinking patterns, will help you determine how much work you need to do on your thinking patterns. (You should have already practiced this with the self-monitoring diaries that you completed in chapters 2 and 6.) To identify your thinking patterns, you need to attend to the content of your thoughts (stream of consciousness). In the situations you record, ask yourself: "What thoughts went through my mind?" Remember to be specific. The more literal you are in recording your thoughts, the better.

It takes some time to learn to analyze your thoughts. This is because thinking patterns become routine and *automatic*. When specific thought patterns become routine, they also become *shorthand* in nature. For example, every time a friend asks you to go to dinner, you think, "What if I have uncontrollable gas during the meal?" In this situation, your next thought might be, "Oh no, I can't," which is shorthand for "Oh no, I can't.

If I go, I may have uncontrollable gas and humiliate myself." Notice the translation required to go from the experienced thought to the underlying meaning. It helps to record your thoughts in the form of statements, not questions ("What if I have gas?" usually means "I will have gas and humiliate myself."). It is also useful to keep in mind that thoughts can occur as words (self-talk) or images, such as picturing yourself expelling smelly gas at a busy restaurant and people turning to look at you. Finally, to help you learn to identify stress-related automatic thoughts, ask yourself the following question when you are recording your thoughts: "What was upsetting me in this situation?" Don't apply logic and reason when answering this question; base your answer on your distressing feelings.

It may help you to think about this using the ABC method. A refers to the *activating event* (the situation that brought on your stress/symptoms); B refers to your *beliefs* or thoughts in the situation; and C refers to the emotional and behavioral *consequences*.

Think back over the past week (or two) and identify a situation in which you either felt stress or had an episode of irritable bowel that you believe was stress related. Take a moment and recall the details of the situation. The more details you can recall the better. Using the following table, write down the situation in the first column. In the second column, write down the thoughts that were associated with the situation. In the third column, write down your feelings.

Situation (What, when, where, who?)	Automatic Thoughts (What were you thinking at the time?)	Feelings (How did it make you feel?)
_____	_____	_____
_____	_____	_____
_____	_____	_____
_____	_____	_____
_____	_____	_____

Self-Analysis

Following the self-monitoring instructions, keep a record for four to five days when you are having symptoms, then sit down and analyze the results. Do you see a tendency toward negative thinking? Are you worrying about how things will work out or your ability to cope? If so, you will need to learn to confront and challenge negative thinking styles.

Changing Your Thinking (Cognitive Restructuring)

Cognitive restructuring is a technical term that psychologists use to refer to the process of changing, or restructuring, your thoughts. In particular, improving coping and quality of life often involves learning how to evaluate situations in a realistic way that helps us, not harms us. It is easy to become overwhelmed and feel like giving up. Pessimism is infectious! Maintaining a realistic optimism is difficult but important. Once you have identified your negative, stress-inducing thoughts, confront them. Challenge your negative thinking. Ask yourself:

- Are there any other ways of thinking about this?
- If I were giving advice to a friend who was thinking this, what would I say?
- If I can't change the situation, how can I live with it?

Cognitive restructuring is difficult to learn, and most people give up on it easily. This is because negative thinking styles are automatic once they set in, and automatic thoughts are more believable. At first, coping thoughts are not very believable. With practice, however, they become more believable. This is particularly true if you can prove yourself wrong.

Psychologists have identified typical thinking styles that are associated with distress. Learning about these styles can also help you alter your thoughts. The following table describes common negative distortions in our thinking.

Negative Thinking Style	Definition
Catastrophizing	The tendency to think in terms of worst-case scenarios. Often experienced as "what if" thoughts.
Black-and-white thinking	Thinking that situations are either all good or all bad, with little in-between.

Magnifying/minimizing	The tendency to overemphasize negative events and under-emphasize positive events.
Selective attention	The tendency to focus only on the negative or stressful aspects of a situation and ignore the positive.
Personalizing	The tendency to think that bad things reflect your character, rather than just luck or circumstances.

There is an important stress reaction for which cognitive restructuring can be helpful to those with irritable bowel. This is the stress caused by irritable bowel symptoms. In our experience, most of this distress is related to upsetting thoughts that you have about your irritable bowel symptoms. It will help if you can confront these negative thoughts directly and build your confidence in coping by reminding yourself that irritable bowel symptoms are modifiable and that the more effort you put into coping, the more likely you will succeed.

Reducing the Stress

Up to this point, we have talked about what you can do to reduce the effects of stress, by calming your body and calming your mind. Equally important, however, is to reduce the stress whenever possible.

You already know that there are two types of stress: controllable and uncontrollable (recall chapter 8). Uncontrollable stress is caused by events about which you can't do anything. The death of a loved one, losing your job, having your house burn down are all examples of uncontrollable stresses. With uncontrollable stresses, you need to accept the stress and minimize its effect on you.

By contrast, controllable stresses include things like being unemployed (you might not be able to control losing your job, but you can try to get another), conflict in a relationship, or being overwhelmed at work. By controllable, we don't mean that you have total control; we do mean that there are things you can do to influence the outcome. You need to take action to help manage controllable stress.

Learning the difference between controllable and uncontrollable stresses is very difficult. You need to ask yourself: "Is there anything I might be able to do about this situation?" or "Does everyone react to this stress the same way, or do other people do something different?" Also, it is helpful to ask a person you trust whether he or she considers your stress issue controllable or not. Often, others can see some action we can take that we are unable to see.

We recommend the following strategies when trying to change the stress in your life:

- Problem solving (brainstorm, evaluate the pros and cons, pick a solution, try it out, and evaluate the outcome)
- Time management (set realistic priorities and limits, and plan for relaxation)
- Assertiveness (broken record and fogging)

Problem Solving

If you are going to work through a problem, do it when you are relatively calm, have some time, and aren't preoccupied with other things. Going to a new surrounding often helps. For instance, you could go to the park on a sunny day, to a favorite coffee shop, or to some other situation that takes you out of your routine. Often, we can think more clearly about a situation when we are removed from it. Be sure to have pen and paper with you.

1. Write down the problem in a clear, brief manner.
2. Write down what you'd like to see happen; what is your realistic goal.
3. Brainstorm. Write down all possible solutions, without evaluating any. Don't worry how silly or unfeasible the solution seems; just get it down on paper.
4. Now go back and consider each possible solution. Carefully think through each one before dismissing it. Be sure to blend and modify as you go through the list.

5. Pick the best solution from the list.
6. Write down the advantages and disadvantages of following through on this solution. You might want to discuss this option with someone you trust to get his or her opinion.
7. Follow through on this solution.
8. Evaluate the outcome of your solution. How did it work?
9. Go back to step 1 if you are not satisfied with the results.

Time Management

A great deal of stress that contributes to irritable bowel results from living a hectic lifestyle in which we cram as much as we can into the limited time we have. As a result, managing our time is extremely important. Time management involves three main tasks: setting realistic goals, prioritizing (which really means deciding that we will *not* get some things done), and building relaxation into our plan.

Sit down with pen and paper and make a list of the tasks you have for the next week. Now consider how much time each will reasonably take (it might be a good idea to multiply your time estimate by 1.5, as most tasks take longer than we plan) and how much time you have. Now make sure you plan in time to eat your meals leisurely and to use relaxation methods.

Assertiveness

Our experience in working with stress issues in general, and stress-related bowel symptoms in particular, is that relationships are a major source of stress. Therefore, we want to give you two useful methods for dealing with difficult people. These are verbal methods that will help you to get your point across without getting angry or pulled into an argument and to deal with negative comments from others. These methods are called *broken record* and *fogging*.

Broken Record

If you want to make a point but don't believe that the person you are talking to wants to hear you, the broken record method will help. In such situations, most people try to explain and justify themselves. So if you say, "I don't think I'll be able to stay late tonight to work" and your boss says, "But I'll only need you for an hour, maybe less. I'm sure you can swing that," you might want to respond by explaining yourself (for example, "But I told my husband I'd get dinner started early tonight"). This is not a great response because it leaves you open for a counterresponse ("Why don't you just get takeout? I know you like Swiss Chalet."). You then need to come back with another explanation. If the other person doesn't really want to hear you, you will usually run out of explanations before he or she runs out of pressuring comments.

To avoid this, use the broken record. This is how it works. First, identify what it is you want to say. Try to keep it simple and polite. Now, like a broken record, repeat the exact same thing (word for word) over and over again, regardless of what the other person says. If you can prepare in advance, think of what you want to say in the most direct way using as few words as possible and in a polite tone. Then just repeat this over and over. Make sure you use exactly the same words and the same tone of voice no matter how many times you repeat it. Resist the temptation to explain more. After three or four repetitions the other person will get the message and stop pressuring you.

Try this with a friend. Set up a role-play situation, in which your friend asks you to deliver a package for him or her. You respond with, "Sorry, but I won't be able to do it." Ask your friend to give you a hard time about this. Once you've tried this once or twice, you'll see how liberating it is.

Fogging

Communication (sending messages) in general and the broken record method in particular would be much easier if the person you were talking to kept silent and listened. Inevitably, however, the other person has something to say, probably something you don't want to hear. You can't just ignore what the other person says, and quite often your response escalates the conflict. People often feel that they are in a no-win situation in these circumstances (you can't say anything, and anything you say will be used against you). Consider the following exchange:

Gail: I have to leave early and the boss needs this in a half hour, so I'll leave it on your desk. Thanks.

Tina: Sorry, but I've got a deadline from Debbie, so I won't be able to do it.

Gail: But I'm sure yours can wait. This is really important and I can't miss my appointment. I know Debbie is out this afternoon, so if you get it to her first thing tomorrow, I'm sure it will be fine.

Tina: I've got a deadline as well, so I won't be able to do it. Debbie gave me two things to do, so I won't have time tomorrow.

Gail: But you can stay late—you said the kids are staying over at your parents.

Tina: Yeah, but I wanted to do some shopping on the way home.

Gail: I heard there is a big sale at the mall starting tomorrow, so why don't you go then?

Tina: I can't go tomorrow—Brian has his game.

Gail: But the games don't start till six. Why are you being so difficult? How can your shopping be more important than this appointment? You know I haven't been feeling well—I thought you were my friend.

Tina: I am your friend. Just leave the memo and I'll try to get to it.

Gail: Thanks, you're a peach.

Tina: No problem. [Inside she is thinking, I'm not a peach; I'm a sucker.]

Does this scenario sound familiar? The situation is typical in that Gail is invested in controlling Tina to solve her own problem. Notice that Tina did okay for the first two comments (she stuck with the broken record). But things went haywire when she started to respond to the specifics of what Gail said. As the conversation continued, the point Tina was trying to make (I have my own deadline) got forgotten and Gail got more pushy, finally questioning the friendship (and implying that Tina was insensitive by comparing her medical problem to going shopping). At this point, Tina caved in and agreed to do the work.

If you step back from this scenario, you can see that Gail had a problem: she couldn't complete her deadline and go to her appointment. Instead of dealing with her boss, she tried to push the problem onto

Tina. She did this because she didn't want to upset her boss. Since her boss holds more power over her than Tina, she probably didn't even give much thought to Tina (since that would make her uncomfortable). All this is quite reasonable, and one can see why she did what she did. However, Tina (you) has the *choice* whether or not she wants to solve Gail's problem. If Tina is able to, then she might simply say in her first reply, "Sure, I can finish this later, don't worry about it." But if she isn't able to accommodate Gail, she has the right to make that choice. Then it is Gail's problem to solve some other way.

How can you avoid falling into this trap? You can use the fogging method. Fogging is the art of agreeing without actually agreeing. Sound confusing? It really isn't. To avoid an escalating conflict in a situation like Tina's, find something in what the person said and acknowledge or agree with it *without agreeing to the behavior the person wants from you*. Also, be sure to use the broken record method each time you respond. Let's go through the previous scenario again, this time using the fogging method.

Gail: I have to leave early and the boss needs this in a half hour, so I'll leave it on your desk. Thanks.

Tina: Sorry, but I've got a deadline from Debbie, so I won't be able to do it.

Gail: But I'm sure yours can wait. This is really important and I can't miss my appointment. I know Debbie is out this afternoon, so if you get yours to her first thing tomorrow, I'm sure it will be fine.

Tina: I understand that it's important and that you can't miss your appointment, but I've got a deadline as well, so I won't be able to do it.

Gail: But you can stay late—you said the kids are staying over at your parents.

Tina: Yeah, that's true, but I've got a deadline as well, so I won't be able to do it.

Gail: But your deadline can't be more important than mine.

Tina: That may be true, but I've got a deadline as well, so I won't be able to do it.

Gail: Why are you being so difficult? You know I haven't been feeling well—I thought you were my friend.

Tina: I can see why you think I'm being difficult, but I've got a deadline as well, so I won't be able to do it.

Gail: Are you sure there is no way you can do it?

Tina: Sorry, but I've got a deadline as well, so I won't be able to do it.

Gail: Okay, I'll see if Bob can do it.

Notice the difference between these two scenarios. In the second, Tina consistently used the broken record, which enabled her to not lose sight of the point she wanted to make and not get dragged into a debate about other points. By using fogging, she was able to respond to Gail in a way that was polite and acknowledged her issues but did not give in to her. Tina was able to choose what to respond to in what Gail said (for example, about being difficult) without getting into other more touchy issues (for example, not being her friend). In our experience, this scenario is realistic in that after using the broken record and fogging four or five times consecutively the other person gets the point. Notice the last thing Gail says is an acknowledgment that she recognizes that Tina is making her own decision (that is, is not allowing Gail to push her problem onto Tina).

These verbal methods (broken record and fogging) take practice before they can be used comfortably. The practice is well worth it, as these methods can eliminate a lot of stress brought on by people who are unreasonable in their demands on you. The following is a form that you can use to keep track of your practicing these methods.

Use this form to keep track of your experiences practicing the broken record and fogging methods. In choosing situations to try out these methods, you might identify an actual event or stage an artificial situation in which you ask someone to act out a role and you respond (we call this role-play). For each situation, put a checkmark under the method you used and rate, using a scale of 1 to 10, how well it worked.

Hint: At first, it might help if you write down what you would like to say for the broken record and keep this handy. Remember to say the same thing over and over, without changing anything. Also, come up with a list of fogging statements that you could use in a variety of situations. Most people find that several stock statements carry them through most situations. Examples of good fogging statements are:

- I can see why you would say that.
- You might be right.
- I can see that you want me to do _____ (whatever).
- I can see your point.

Situation	Broken Record	Fogging
_____	_____	_____
_____	_____	_____
_____	_____	_____
_____	_____	_____
_____	_____	_____

Matching Method to Symptom

While it is true that each person is unique and must find his or her own effective stress management strategies, it is also true that certain methods can be best applied for certain symptoms. There are two ways to look at this: the nature of the stress that causes your symptoms and the nature of the symptoms themselves. If the source of your stress is external to yourself (that is, your work environment or conflict with family or friends), focus on the strategies in the "Reducing the Stress" section. If, however, the main source of your stress is internal (your tendency to worry or catastrophize), focus on the "Calming Your Mind" section. If your main stress is the effect that the symptoms themselves have on you once they start, the section "Calming Your Body" is for you.

Also consider the nature of your symptoms. Recall that the primary symptoms of irritable bowel include abdominal pain, change in bowel habits (increased frequency and looseness, or alternating periods of constipation), mucus, abdominal bloating, and sensations of incomplete rectal emptying. Relaxation and imagery methods are often very effective for managing pain. Similarly, relaxation methods and cognitive restructuring help a great deal with altered bowel habits. Mucus is usually not of great concern to people with irritable bowel, but if it is, it is usually due to excessive worry about it. In this case, cognitive restructuring is most useful. Similarly, although not of great medical consequence, abdominal bloating can be very worrisome to people, especially since the degree of bloating can be quite marked. Again, cognitive restructuring can be the method of choice to deal with this specific situation. Finally, sensations of incomplete rectal emptying are usually related to increased attention focused on the rectal area. Imagery and cognitive restructuring can be very useful in distracting your attention away from the sensations in this area of your body, and in this way reducing the intensity of this symptom.

Putting It All Together

We covered a lot of material in this chapter. To benefit from it, you will need to review it carefully. We encourage you to reread this chapter. Only by trial and error will you discover how the methods described in this chapter will work for you, and which of them is best suited to managing your symptoms. We've provided all the ingredients; it is up to you to combine them into a stew. As with food, these methods must fit your taste (not to mention your lifestyle). Above all, you need to know this about stress management methods: No one method has been shown to be the best for managing stress. The best method is the one that makes sense to you, that you can learn to do well, that suits your personality and life situations, and that you can follow through with. Don't expect these methods to work magically. They are, however, as a group, the most effective stress management strategies that are available for managing irritable bowel symptoms. Remember to have fun and enjoy these methods!

10

What Do I Do about the Pain?

Pain is the most common symptom of irritable bowel and the symptom most likely to cause a person to seek medical attention. This is because we all interpret pain as a sign that something is seriously wrong with our bodies. Also, most of us believe that the intensity of pain reflects the seriousness of harm. However, while your pain can be severe and is very real (not just "in your head"), it is not causing any damage to your bowel (it hurts but does not harm).

It is important for you to understand that we are not telling you that your pain is not real. It is just that your pain does not signal danger or damage. At our clinic, we recently completed a study of the pain experience of individuals with irritable bowel and compared it to the pain experienced by those with Crohn's disease, an inflammatory bowel disease. This study was clear in showing that the pain experience of those with irritable bowel was every bit as severe as the pain experience of those with Crohn's disease. There was only one measure that showed a difference between the two groups: social support. On this measure, those with Crohn's disease reported more social support than did those with irritable bowel. This tells us that the suffering of those with irritable bowel can actually be greater than of those with Crohn's.

The pain is the same, but those with irritable bowel get less social support from others. So we understand that the pain is real, but that it is not a sign of harm; it is a sign of hurt.

Making the distinction between hurt and harm is very important in pain management. You can learn to live with hurt. The pain will make you feel bad, but it does not mean that any damage is being done to the bowel or that your symptoms will lead to a serious bowel disease (such as colitis or bowel cancer). But how do you learn to live with pain?

In learning to manage pain, you first need to change how you view the pain and the things that you say to yourself while you are in pain. The automatic reaction to pain is to become alarmed. After all, pain is one of the body's alarm systems. If you become familiar enough with your pain (so you know the difference between regular hurt and unexplained symptoms that might indicate harm) and are adequately reassured that the pain is not harmful, you can learn to remain calm and work with, not against, pain. Critical to doing this is distinguishing hurt from harm.

Hurt versus Harm

Hurt refers to the experience of pain that is not damaging. For instance, take the muscle pain experienced after a workout. This is clearly pain, but it does not cause any damage.

By *harm* we refer to pain that is an indication of damage being done. If you've just undergone surgery, pain around the incision when you move is often a sign to stop so that you avoid damage, such as by tearing the stitches or staples open. The pain associated with irritable bowel hurts but it does not harm. It is okay to experience this pain. In fact, by making it okay (a decision you make) you will find that you can work with your pain, not against it.

Our experience in treating people with chronic pain is that after successful treatment, the individual says, "You know, I still have the pain, but it is not as bad as before and it doesn't upset me as it used to. Now I manage the pain, rather than it managing me."

How do you decide what pain is hurtful and not harmful? This first requires a proper diagnosis of your condition as irritable bowel (see chapters 1 and 2). Then you need to ask yourself: "Is this pain familiar? Is it the typical pain I experience with my irritable bowel?" If it is, then recognize the pain as hurt not harm (even if the pain is intense and continues to alarm you). If your pain is new or changes dramatically, then you may need to consult your doctor to help evaluate whether the pain reflects hurt or harm.

Initially, you should see your doctor about whether your pain is due to irritable bowel or some other problem or disease. There are nine things that your doctor will want to know about the pain. These nine things will also help you to better identify what you may be doing that will make the pain better or worse.

Nine Things to Know about Your Pain

1. Where is the pain?
2. Does the pain go anywhere else, such as the back, shoulders, and so on?
3. What does the pain feel like? Common terms used to describe pain include: *sharp like a knife*, *burning*, *gnawing*, and *cramping*.
4. How long does the pain last?
5. Have you noticed anything that reduces the pain? For instance, lying down, drinking milk or taking an antacid, rubbing your abdomen, or using an ice pack or hot pack?
6. Have you noticed anything that worsens or triggers the pain? For instance, eating, bending over, lifting heavy objects, bowel motions, and so on?
7. What were you doing when the pain started?
8. Has the pain ever wakened you from a deep sleep?
9. Have you ever had pain of a similar quality or pattern in the past, even if it was some years ago?

How to Manage the Pain

Pain is a very personal experience. People will not experience the same level of pain in response to the same level of stimulation. Also, under different circumstances people will experience different pain levels to the same stimulation. We have all heard of situations where someone has hurt himself or herself but experienced little pain. The athlete who injures him or herself during a game often keeps playing without feeling pain. But when the game ends, the pain starts. If that same injury resulted from a car accident or after you fell down stairs, you can bet that the pain would be worse. The actual damage might not be worse, but the experience of pain would be.

Pain intensity (as perceived) is influenced by attention and distress. The more you focus on the pain and the more it upsets you, the more intense the pain will feel. It works the other way, too: the less you focus on the pain and the less it upsets you, the less pain you experience. Only *you* experience the intensity of your pain; therefore, it is important to understand the factors that will influence how intensely you will experience your pain. Understanding this will help you to better manage your pain.

Pain can vary in its intensity depending on your state of mind. If you are a person who spends your time monitoring your body for symptoms (see the section on somatizing and body vigilance in chapter 12), then you will tend to experience pain more intensely than other people. This is because you focus more intensely on your body than do others and probably get easily alarmed if you experience something unfamiliar.

If you are the type of person who tends to ignore what is going on in your body, you may feel less pain. This is similar to the football player who breaks a bone in his foot during the fourth quarter of a crucial game. Because he is so focused on winning, he barely notices the pain, yet he needs crutches to leave the locker room after the game. If that same individual had the same injury while doing something less intense, he would immediately find the pain intolerable. The injury in both instances is the same, yet the experience of the pain is quite different. By learning techniques that help distract you from—or be less aware of—the pain, you will learn to manage your pain without always resorting to pain medications.

Pain Management Strategies

There are three steps to controlling pain: controlling your thoughts, controlling your body, and controlling your behavior.

Controlling Your Thoughts

This strategy is similar to the general coping strategies covered in chapter 9. You need to talk yourself through pain episodes. We need to emphasize again that the normal response of the body to pain is to go into alarm mode. Pain produces an automatic reaction, just like a reflex. When something causes you pain, you immediately focus your attention on the pain and prepare your body for action, increasing muscle tension. When you cannot take action to alleviate the pain right away, you become distressed. This increases your body tension and focuses you even more clearly on your pain. This is what we call the *pain cycle*. Your job is to prevent your body from automatically going into alarm mode when your irritable bowel pain begins.

To control your thoughts, you need to:

- *Understand what is happening.* You will need to tell yourself, over and over, that the pain is not a sign of something wrong, but is a part of your irritable bowel (it hurts but it doesn't harm). It might help to think about the pain caused by a charley horse. We've all experienced a charley horse in one of our muscles, such as the calf muscle. This pain is clearly intense, but it signals no real danger. We stretch out the muscle and the pain eventually goes away. What would happen if we couldn't stretch out the muscle? The pain would continue. This is what is happening in your bowel. The bowel is a large tubelike muscle, and when it spasms or goes into a charley horse, you can't straighten it out. You need to endure the pain and relax the muscle so that the spasm (charley horse) goes away. Thinking about your bowel pain as a charley horse may help to convince you that the pain, while intense, is not serious.
- *Accept chronic pain.* You will need to make friends with your pain. Yes, you heard us correctly. Since your normal bowel produces pain, then the pain is normal for you. This is why you may need to consider some pain medication and why you need to stop the pain cycle.
- *Talk yourself through the pain.* When you are in pain, you will automatically become upset and focused on the pain. You will need to work hard to talk yourself through this. Most people find

that they benefit from self-statements that keep things in perspective. Tell yourself things such as:

> The pain scares me, but I know there is really nothing wrong.
> Don't worry about the pain, just relax and focus on something else.
> I've had this same pain many times before and it always goes away after a while.
> The more I focus on the pain, the worse it is.

Controlling Your Body

Pain is an alarm signal, and the body, like a fire department, responds to all alarms, even false ones. The body's response to alarm is to increase muscle tension, heart rate, and blood pressure and to secrete stress hormones. If you want to reduce your pain, you will need to learn to control this bodily response. The best way to do this is with relaxation techniques.

Review and practice the relaxation techniques presented in chapter 9. Remember that it is very difficult to use relaxation techniques when you are in pain (it's like trying to stay calm when your house is on fire), so master them when you are calm, before episodes of pain. You will need to be patient and not give up on relaxation.

Controlling Your Behavior

Because your pain hurts but does not harm, it helps to do things other than focusing on the pain. Distracting yourself is very useful. Do some housework, gardening, or some other physical activity that occupies your mind. If there's an opportunity to read, do so, or you might find it helpful to talk with someone. Doing something productive is also helpful in controlling behavior. Not only is it distracting, but the sense of accomplishment when you finish is uplifting as well.

Minimizing certain behaviors can influence your pain. First, avoid isolating yourself. Isolation not only encourages you to focus on your pain, it is depressing, which increases suffering. Second, avoid overrelying on medication. As we discussed earlier, medication can be a useful part of your treatment, but do not expect it to cure you. Even if you find medication helpful, you will still need to find other ways of managing your pain.

Pain Medications

Many people with irritable bowel try medications to relieve pain. There are two types of pain medications: narcotic painkillers that are very effective for acute and short-term pain and medications that appear to modify the pain over the longer term and are more effective for chronic pain.

Narcotic painkillers should never be used for the abdominal pain of irritable bowel. These drugs are addictive and negatively affect the gut. They tend to cause constipation and increased abdominal contractions or spasms that actually worsen the pain. What's more, this side effect persists longer than the painkilling effect of the medication. This leads to a vicious cycle for the person who seeks increasing doses of the painkiller in the mistaken belief that after receiving "enough" medication, the pain will go away. Unfortunately, what usually happens is that the pain is only eased temporarily. It then returns, often with increased intensity due to the increased bowel contractions and spasms caused by the drug. Some individuals become addicted to painkillers because they can never receive enough medication to relieve the pain.

Fortunately, there is a better approach to managing pain with medications, especially if you continue to have frequent and recurrent pain despite practicing techniques to ease the intensity of the pain.

Antidepressants

Antidepressants are a group of drugs that have a beneficial side effect for many people with irritable bowel: they ease chronic pain. When antidepressants are used for chronic pain, they are usually prescribed at much lower doses than those used for treating depression. Your doctor has to prescribe these drugs, so you will have to discuss with him or her which drug is best for you. Other medical problems may make antidepressants inappropriate or potentially dangerous.

If your doctor agrees that an antidepressant drug may be helpful for you, consider these points:

- Antidepressants work best for chronic pain.
- Antidepressants are taken daily, usually at night with the dose gradually increased every four to seven days until the pain eases. They do not have an immediate effect.

Like all medications, antidepressants do have side effects, and you must be regularly monitored by your doctor while taking them. Still, many people with irritable bowel tolerate antidepressants well. Because the dosage is often much lower than the dose needed to treat depression, these medications can be taken for prolonged periods to achieve good pain control.

Antispasm Drugs

Another group of medications used to manage irritable bowel pain are antispasm drugs that decrease the contractions and spasms of the bowel. These drugs have limited usefulness for many people with irritable bowel, but some individuals find them helpful for episodes of bowel spasm. Antispasm drugs have to be prescribed, so you will have to see your doctor about whether or not one of them may be helpful for your pain. Because these drugs decrease the contractions of the bowel to reduce pain, they can have other side effects such as worsening constipation symptoms.

New Drugs

Medical research is also leading to the development of new drugs designed specifically to treat patients with irritable bowel. These new drugs have been developed to help treat abdominal pain along with other bowel symptoms such as diarrhea and constipation. Your doctor will know about these drugs, and she can help you decide if they may be right for your pain. Be sure you take the correct medication. For instance, if you have diarrhea along with abdominal pain, your condition will worsen (especially your diarrhea) if you take the medication that helps abdominal pain and constipation.

If you find medication helpful, you should also try pain management techniques such as those discussed in this chapter. You shouldn't rely on medication alone to resolve your pain completely.

Other Sources of Pain

Some types of pain cannot be effectively treated with medications or coping techniques. For instance, if you review your symptoms diary from chapter 2 and find that there rarely seems to be any aggravating or relieving factors to your pain, it is likely you have a condition called *chronic functional abdominal pain*, rather than irritable bowel. This condition usually requires expert advice and intensive therapy that is beyond the scope of this book. Still, you might find that some of the techniques in this chapter and chapter 9 will help you manage your pain better.

Finally, there are people who suffer from irritable bowel who have a past history of sexual and/or physical abuse. These people often have severe pain as part of their symptoms. If this is your situation, it is important to acknowledge that sexual abuse has happened and to seek professional help for the abuse. It is unlikely that you will be able to properly manage your pain and other bowel symptoms until you have addressed the unresolved psychological pain and injury that results from this abuse. We encourage you to speak to your doctor or seek help from a psychologist or psychiatrist or other mental health therapist experienced in treating people who have been abused.

11

Are You Ready? Making Change Happen

It is obvious that managing irritable bowel involves making behavior changes. We have made many suggestions, both having to do with eating and with identifying and managing stress. The scientific literature supports us in recommending these behavior changes because they often lead to significant improvement in irritable bowel symptoms and quality of life. We are also aware that changing behavior is not easy, however. Many people would agree with the following statement: "I am able to start something new, can keep doing it for four weeks or eight weeks or sometimes even twelve weeks, but then I slip and end up back at the place where I started."

The fact is, it is easier to start a new behavior than it is to keep up this behavior (or behaviors). If this is true for you, you might be reassured to know that it is true for most people. That is why it is so difficult for people to stop smoking, lose weight, or exercise on a regular basis. It can be even more challenging when you are trying to change several behaviors at one time, which is likely if you have discovered that both food and stress trigger your irritable bowel. Even though your irritable bowel symptoms can be a source of major distress in your life, you may find that the changes we recommend in this book are harder to implement than you would like.

Nowhere is the struggle to maintain behavior change more common than with healthy eating or weight management. Being overweight or obese is a problem for millions of North Americans. The majority of overweight people would like to lose weight and eat healthy, and many have tried a number of diets and exercise plans to do so. But most of these people are unable to keep the weight off. Some even regain more weight than they lose.

So we are left with a situation in which a person wants to do something new, tries it, sees that it helps, but cannot keep the behavior going. In this chapter, we want to help you understand why this pattern is so common and how you can avoid it. It really comes down to motivation. The bottom line is that people do the things that they are strongly motivated to do. The more motivated you are, the more effort you put into something and the more likely you will keep at it until you achieve it. We've all heard stories of the marathon runner who, despite "hitting the wall," keeps going because of determination and will.

You need to appreciate that motivation is based not only on the positive things that achieving something brings but also on the negative things. So you might discover that eliminating certain foods from your diet will improve your irritable bowel symptoms. But what if you are an emotional eater and these foods bring you comfort in times of stress? If you eliminate these foods from your diet, your irritable bowel improves, but you have lost a method of managing your stress. What we are trying to say is that there are advantages and disadvantages to almost everything. It is the balance between the advantages and disadvantages, as well as your willingness to accept the disadvantages, that determines true motivation.

Take emotional eating as an example. The majority of people who are emotional eaters find that high-fat, calorie-dense foods are more comforting than healthier foods. Emotional eaters also tend to overeat when distressed. When they eat enough food to calm them emotionally, they may experience irritable bowel symptoms. If they want to reduce these symptoms, there are good reasons to avoid eating large amounts of high-fat, high-calorie foods and other foods that provoke irritable bowel symptoms. Eating foods that cause fewer irritable bowel symptoms could also have disadvantages, however. We often hear people tell us that irritable bowel–friendly foods require extra preparation, may be harder to find in grocery stores or specialty shops, cost more, and are not familiar to others. Since we like to eat with others, choosing foods that do not fit socially may add to the challenge of managing irritable bowel.

To maintain a behavior, motivation has to be high. For motivation to be high, we have to want the changes and be willing to accept the disadvantages of a change. Keeping the disadvantages in mind is important because healthy behaviors often require effort, and the effort does not diminish over time. For example, it is more expensive to buy healthy foods than unhealthy foods. It costs money and takes time to join and go to an exercise club. These costs will remain the same or even increase (as in the price of a health club membership) over time.

Consider the following question: "Would you like to have a new Mercedes Benz?" You can't really answer this question without being aware of the costs. If the question is "Would you like to have a new Mercedes Benz for $5,000?" many of you would say yes. If I were to ask "Would you like to have this new Mercedes Benz for $5,000 if I will throw in all the service visits for five years?" more of you would say yes. But if I were to ask, "Would you like this Mercedes Benz for $75,000 if all service visits will cost at least $1,000?" almost all of you would say no. Motivation is not just about wanting something; it is also about being willing to accept the costs. If this book helps you, it will be helpful because it will guide you to make behavior changes. To make these changes last, however, you must be motivated to continue your new behavior patterns.

It may be interesting for you to note that normal psychological functioning also works against change. This is because it is human nature to prefer things that are predictable and routine. It's easier that way. We don't have to put as much thought into it. If, for example, the rules of the road were that we drive on the right-hand side Mondays, Wednesdays, and Fridays, and the left-hand side on Tuesdays, Thursdays, and Saturdays, and on Sundays the side you drive on depends on whether it is the first, third or fifth Sunday as opposed to the second or fourth, driving would be a nightmare. Since we always drive on the right-hand side, we don't have to think about it and can direct our attention to other things. So much of our behavior becomes habit. Changing habits requires attention, and attention is limited. This applies to the behaviors associated with irritable bowel symptoms: if these behaviors are habits, they will be difficult to change and will require focused attention.

As humans, we prefer to take the path of least resistance. So if there is a simpler way of doing something, the simple way will be chosen. It is much simpler to drive through a fast-food restaurant where everyone in the car can choose their own meals than it is to prepare the food at home, trying to please everyone with one meal. It is also human nature for us to focus on the short term rather than the long term. Most of us choose behaviors that bring short-term gain even if they result in long-term pain. However, healthy behavior often requires short-term pain to bring long-term gain. Investing in a retirement savings plan is a good example of long-term thinking. Most everyone could make good use of the money right now, but we know that if we save for the future that money will increase in value through compound interest and time. This is easier said than done, however.

By this point in the book, you have a pretty good idea about the kind of changes that we are talking about. We have asked you to assess yourself with regard to the things you eat and the stress issues in your life and how they affect your irritable bowel symptoms. Based on this assessment we hope you are able to identify the types of changes that you think are important for you to make to manage your irritable bowel. You are unique and your own person; therefore, you need a plan that is specifically tailored to you. In the chart on page 163, you can outline your plan by writing out the changes that you think are important for you to make to improve your irritable bowel. Identify changes you want to make in your diet and in managing stress.

Rate Your Readiness

Now you have some idea of the kinds of changes that you want to make. Next, ask yourself what the advantages and disadvantages of these changes are. Why do you want to do these things? How will they help you? What will be hard about these changes?

SETTING A RELEVANT GOAL

Based on my self-assessment, the following changes to my eating patterns will help my irritable bowel symptoms (refer back to chapter 6, where you completed your food and symptom record):

What I eat:

_____

_____

How much I eat:

_____

_____

When I eat:

_____

_____

Other changes to my diet:

_____

_____

Based on my self-assessment, here are some things I need to do differently to better manage my stress and reduce irritable bowel symptoms (refer back to chapter 8, where you completed your stress diary):

What I need to do that I am not doing:

_____

_____

What I need to do more of:

_____

_____

What I need to do less of:

_____

_____

Other changes to manage stress:

_____

_____

You can now evaluate your level of motivation. You have some idea of the specific changes that are relevant to you (after all, you identified them), why you would want to make these changes, and why these changes will be difficult. Put all this together and select from the following statements the one that best describes your current intention to change. Don't pick the statement that you think you should select, or that you think others would want you to select. If you start with an honest assessment of your readiness to change, you can avoid setting yourself up for failure and can gain the maximum value from this workbook.

1. I am ready to make changes to my diet and to practice stress management techniques.
2. I am thinking about making changes to my diet and practicing stress management techniques, and may follow through in the next month.
3. I am thinking about making changes to my diet and practicing stress management techniques, and may follow through in the next six months.
4. I am not thinking about making changes to my diet or practicing stress management techniques, and won't for the next six months.

Notice that we have lumped together diet and stress management. We do this just for convenience. You might be more ready to change one behavior than the other. Feel free to fill this out for each behavior separately if you think it would be helpful. Readiness is very strongly influenced by many different factors, so break it down as specifically as you would like. Here's a good example: Many people have no problem eating healthy breakfasts. If people are unhealthy in their breakfast meal, it is usually because they do not eat enough, or they skip breakfast entirely. The evening meal, or snacking in the evening, can be very different: most people have difficulty making healthy selections and eat too much. So readiness for healthy eating can depend on the time of day or even the day of the week (compare Monday evening to Friday evening). This is why it is important for you to get a sense of the changes that are critical for you to make. If you can change the key behaviors, you will have a better chance of controlling your irritable bowel.

If you chose statement 1, you are ready to take action to manage your irritable bowel. In that case, this workbook is ideal for you. The chapters are written to provide you with information, but mostly to guide you through hands-on techniques that will allow you to determine the pattern of your symptoms, identify the things that trigger your symptoms, and, based on this, take action to control your symptoms. We cover a lot of material in this workbook, so go slowly. You might find it useful to read a chapter through once, to get an idea of the scope of topics covered and the range of things that you will be asked to do. Then read the chapter again, going slowly and practicing the strategies. The techniques in this workbook are presented in what we call a "cafeteria" approach. By this we mean that you should feel free to pick and choose specific techniques that feel right and work for you. This will allow you to match the techniques to your symptoms, personality, and lifestyle.

If you picked statement 2, you are getting ready for change. You should find this workbook helpful in providing information and giving you some ideas about how to change. We recommend that you try the techniques we suggest, but don't be surprised if you're not fully prepared to put in all the effort and commitment to following through with them. You should try them as a way of helping you determine the costs and benefits of putting the strategies from this workbook into practice. If, after you have gone through the workbook, you decide that you are ready to commit yourself, it may be helpful to go through the workbook again to get the maximum value of the techniques.

If you selected statement 3, you are only thinking about change but are not ready to commit yourself. This workbook will be useful as a source of information and as a reference if you decide that you do want to try to change. Don't expect big results from anything you try if you selected this statement. In order for the workbook to make a significant impact on your symptoms, you've got to be willing to persevere with the techniques; this requires an upfront commitment. If you're not ready for this commitment, you're just not ready. Don't beat yourself up for this. It may help if you write a list of the advantages and disadvantages of using this workbook, and a list of the negatives of having irritable bowel. Only when people experience significant distress about having irritable bowel and see more advantages than disadvantages of trying to control symptoms through diet and stress management are they able to commit energy and effort into a workbook such as this one.

If you chose statement 4, it is unlikely that you will read all of this book or follow the instructions. If someone else has suggested that you read this book, you may be doing it for that person and not for yourself. If this describes you, don't expect much from this workbook. The most you would get out of it is information that may help you decide to change at some point in the future.

If you are interested in trying out the strategies for coping that we outline in this workbook, there are a few other tips we can give you that may help. Once people start the process of change, which as we've seen is best when motivation is high, two things need to happen. The first is that your confidence in doing the new behaviors needs to increase if the behavior is likely to stay changed. People who have confidence in their abilities will persevere in difficult situations. People who have little confidence find it more difficult to keep going when things become challenging. So try to build your confidence by practicing and getting comfortable using the strategies in different situations. A good rule of thumb is to *not* try to do something new unless you can say with 80 percent confidence that you truly believe that you can keep the behavior going for at least six months. If you do not have this much confidence, break the behavior down into smaller steps, or find another behavior where you have 80 percent confidence. Nothing builds confidence like success and the more success you have the more confidence you have. So don't bite off more than you can chew!

The second thing that is critical to long-term change is awareness of barriers and temptations. These are the things that get in the way of you doing the healthy behavior and the things that tempt you. We encourage you to identify these barriers and temptations and to develop a plan ahead of time for how you will handle them if and when they arise. If you have a plan, it is so much easier to cope when you find yourself in these situations. So when you run into a barrier, write it down and try to think of a way around it. Also, when you find that you are tempted to slip, write what the temptations are and come up with a plan to deal with them. The following chart will help you with this.

1. List the barriers to change that you have experienced or might experience. Then think of how you can overcome these barriers and write them down as well:

Barrier	**How to Overcome the Barrier**
_____	_____
_____	_____
_____	_____
_____	_____
_____	_____
_____	_____
_____	_____

2. List the temptations that make it hard for you to change. Then think of how you can overcome these temptations and write them down as well:

Temptation	**How to Overcome the Temptation**
_____	_____
_____	_____
_____	_____
_____	_____
_____	_____
_____	_____
_____	_____

Here are a few other recommendations to help you maintain the changes that you find helpful in this book:

- Expect setbacks. No one is perfect, and most of us slip. If you can accept that this will happen and have a plan for getting back on track, it will help greatly. Above all, avoid guilt.
- Find people who will support you in your new behavior. It is much easier to keep with a behavior if we are associating with others who share our commitment.

- Make a commitment to change and make this commitment public. Don't be afraid to set goals, just make them realistic. Once you have a realistic goal, tell someone. It has been shown that if you make a public commitment you are more likely to follow through than if you keep the commitment to yourself.

Good luck!

12

Irritable Bowel Is Not
My Only Worry

Irritable bowel is a significant management problem in its own right. Unfortunately, some people suffer from additional problems, both medical and psychological. In this chapter, we will address two additional psychological problems that are commonly seen in people with irritable bowel: a general pattern of worry and anxiety over one's health and significant emotional distress, such as clinical depression. The first of these issues can be called *somatic preoccupation* (*soma* means the body); the second, *psychopathology*. It is not our intent to provide a detailed method for how to treat these problems. We will explain them, however, and make general suggestions about how to deal with them.

Somatic Preoccupation

For most of us, our health is something we take for granted. This is easily observed by considering the high-risk behaviors most of us engage in on a regular basis, such as smoking, excess drinking, eating high-fat diets, getting too much sun exposure, putting off a physical examination with our doctor, driving without seatbelts, driving above the speed limit, and so on. For others, however, what is going on inside the body and what could happen to their body is a major source of worry and upset. Often, this is because these people have had significant negative experiences in their lives that remind them of how unstable life can be (the multiple sclerosis patient who can only get around with a cane or the relative diagnosed with cancer). Some people, however, have had no significant medical problems and yet remain focused on their health. These people are prone to worry about any body sensation that is unexpected. We refer to these people as *somatically preoccupied*. That is, these people are overly focused on their bodies and being ill. There is overlap between those with irritable bowel and those with somatic preoccupation. Because the bowel is easily affected by stress and because those who are somatically preoccupied are easily stressed, the somatically preoccupied person can develop irritable bowel more easily than someone who is generally unconcerned about his or her health or who denies even strong bodily sensations (for example, the person who tries to convince himself that he's having indigestion, not a heart attack).

We all are aware of our bodies, but mostly we focus on our bodies only when we experience a sensation that is unexpected and uncomfortable. Because people who are somatically preoccupied spend too much time focused on their bodies, they are aware of sensations that have no real significance and are not perceived by others. This is a problem, because as one focuses attention internally on the body, the strength of body sensations increases. You learned this when you were practicing relaxation strategies. In this case, you were becoming aware of tension so you could reduce it. The opposite can also happen, however. If when you focused on your body it frightened you, it would be a negative rather than a positive experience.

Try this for yourself: As you are reading this, stop and focus on the sensations in your feet, where they are resting on the ground (take fifteen to twenty seconds to do this now). Now focus on the sensations in your fingers. Now the sensations in your neck. Notice that as you move your attention from one part of your body to the other the sensations in the body part you are focusing on become stronger. Now take a moment to focus your attention inward to your body. Starting at the top of your head, scan your body down to the tips of your toes. Imagine that your attention is like a spotlight that you can shine on your body. Spend a minute doing this and identify the part of your body that is most uncomfortable. You'll be surprised to find out that when you do this you will almost always be able to identify an uncomfortable sensation in one part of your body or another. Now focus in on this sensation. Clear your mind of any other thought and zero in on this discomfort. Notice that the sensation gets stronger.

Those of you who are not somatically preoccupied will notice a slight increase in the strength of the sensation, but it will quickly fade as your attention returns to other things. Those of you with a tendency to be somatically preoccupied will have more trouble switching your attention away from this sensation. You might even experience a slight increase in feelings of anxiety. Because you have done this in an artificial manner (following these instructions), the sensations are likely to be mild and easily dismissed. However, if this happened spontaneously while you were going about your day, the sensations would be more intense and harder to dismiss. People differ in their attention to bodily sensations; that is, in what we call *body vigilance*. Those who are somatically preoccupied tend to be very highly vigilant.

Body vigilance is one key psychological ingredient in somatic preoccupation. The other is a tendency toward catastrophizing, a term mentioned in chapter 9. Catastrophizing is the tendency to think in terms of worst-case, or catastrophic, scenarios. Those who are somatically preoccupied find it easy to imagine the worst case with their health. For example, they might think that they are developing a serious disease (cancer) if they begin feeling unwell.

Treating somatic preoccupation can be difficult because it often is such a long-standing pattern for the individual that it is the only way he or she has ever thought. In fact, there are psychiatric conditions called *hypochondriasis* and *somatization disorder* that refer to extreme degrees of this condition (more on this later). Regarding somatic preoccupation, three treatment strategies can be suggested: reducing body stress, cognitive restructuring (changing your thinking), and medical management.

Reducing Body Stress

Chronic tension directly feeds body vigilance because it produces stronger body sensations that can be focused on and interpreted catastrophically. Take your left hand, make a fist, and squeeze very tightly. Hold your hand in this position until you start to feel a dull ache; it shouldn't take too long. This pain is very real, hard to ignore, and yet is insignificant. It conveys no risk to your health whatsoever. Yet, we know from chapter 10 that pain is the body's alarm system and that it is difficult to ignore. Learning to relax can be very effective in reducing the tendency to overfocus on the body by reducing physical sensations. You should read chapter 8 to learn a few relaxation exercises.

Cognitive Restructuring

It is essential to convince yourself that the sensations you are catastrophizing about are not significant. This is much easier said than done. Follow the cognitive restructuring methods presented in chapter 9 to help you. It is particularly helpful to establish a series of self-statements to help you reduce both hypervigilance and catastrophizing. We recommend regular practice using the following self-statements:

- I know I tend to worry about my health, but I need to get over it.
- Don't worry about that, just relax and focus on something else.
- I've had this same worry many times before and it always turns out to be nothing.
- The less I worry about it, the less it will bother me.

Any other statement that you think would be helpful to reduce vigilance and catastrophic thinking should be added to this list.

Medical Management

One of the characteristics of those with somatic preoccupation is a strong need for reassurance that nothing is wrong. The best, and often the only, place to get this reassurance is from a physician. Yet, repeated trips to your physician about fears that are dismissed can quickly become frustrating for both you and your physician, as you both are busy. Another problem is the tendency of physicians to use medical investigations to reassure people. This often increases, rather than decreases, worry and upset. For instance, your physician might say, "I don't think there is anything to worry about, but just to be sure, I'll send you for an X-ray" (with the expectation that a negative X-ray will settle you). However, the somatically preoccupied person is likely to think, "I knew something was wrong, he's just saying not to worry to ease the blow. He wouldn't send me for an X-ray if he didn't think there was something wrong." An additional psychological fact needs to be noted. Reassurance to reduce anxiety can be effective, but it wears off very quickly. The person might feel good leaving the doctor's office, but by the next day his or her concerns are back. We see people who are almost addicted to reassurance. Related to this is the tendency to seek additional medical opinions. Because medicine involves a significant amount of judgment on the part of your doctor, if you consult with five doctors about the same problem, you will hear different opinions. This could reflect different ways of saying the same thing or different interpretations. Nonetheless, this can reinforce the anxiety and somatic preoccupation.

To avoid this, we recommend that you find a physician whom you can trust, one who you believe takes you seriously and is concerned about you. Next, you and your physician should establish a set schedule of medical appointments (for example, every four weeks or so; the exact frequency should be worked on an individual basis between you and your doctor). Between appointments, you should cope *on your own*, using the previously mentioned strategies. At the next scheduled appointment, you should voice any concerns that you have, and your physician should provide medical feedback. Consults with other doctors should be minimized, as should medical tests. Only if your doctor, not you, believes a consult or investigation is necessary should it take place (this is why you need to trust your doctor). This can be very effective since you know that you will see your doctor soon and he or she will listen to you and take you seriously. It also works for your doctor since he or she knows what to expect and shouldn't feel that you are overusing the medical system just for reassurance.

Psychopathology

While some people experience irritable bowel in the context of a general tendency to worry about their health (somatic preoccupation), others experience irritable bowel in the context of significant emotional disorders (such as clinical depression). Fortunately, this applies to relatively few people with irritable bowel. Also, most of those who have overlying emotional disorders are diagnosed with mild adjustment disorders, either with an anxious or depressed mood and not serious psychiatric difficulties. Some people, however, have coexisting emotional disorders serious enough to require treatment. The purpose of this section is to outline the most common emotional disorders seen with irritable bowel. In this chapter we will not talk about chronic abdominal pain associated with past sexual abuse (see chapter 11 for more information on coping with past sexual abuse).

If you suspect that you have any of the following emotional disorders, we strongly recommend that you seek help from a licensed mental health practitioner, preferably a psychiatrist or psychologist. Your family doctor might be a good person to discuss this with; often he or she can recommend someone to you. The emotional disorders to look out for include depression, anxiety disorders, and substance abuse disorders.

Depression

We all get sad from time to time, and having a chronic condition like irritable bowel can wear away at your optimism and cheer. Sometimes, however, sadness dominates and becomes a serious problem in itself. This is what we refer to as *clinical depression*. It can be difficult to distinguish normal periods of sadness (the blues) from clinical depression, especially in those who have medical symptoms or for whom depressing events have recently occurred (for example, loss of a job, divorce, and so on). It is often helpful to get feedback from a loved one, your family doctor, or a psychologist or psychiatrist if you think your sadness might be problematic. Clinical depression is likely if your sadness is intense, long lasting, and interferes with your ability to function.

The following are some of the signs to look for if you are concerned that you may be depressed. Place a check mark in each box that applies to you. If you check two or more boxes, you might want to seek professional help or talk to your family doctor about seeking help.

☐ *Sad mood*: Most of the time, for the past two weeks or more you have been feeling sad, down, and blue. Check here ☐ if this sadness has been present for most of the past six months. Check here ☐ if your mood stays down even if something pleasant happens.

☐ *Sleep problems*: Your sleep has been abnormal. Check here ☐ if you are sleeping less than normal (at least two or more hours less sleep most nights); check here ☐ if you are sleeping more than normal. Sleep problems include not being able to get to sleep, not being able to stay asleep, waking early and not being able to get back to sleep, and not feeling rested after sleep.

☐ *Appetite problems*: You have not been eating normally. Check here ☐ if you are eating more than normal; check here ☐ if you are eating less (if you have lost weight as a result of losing your appetite, check here ☐—don't check this box if you are on a weight-loss diet).

☐ *Energy problems*: You are tired all the time. Check here ☐ if you have lost your interest in things; check here ☐ if you have lost your motivation to do things.

☐ *Thinking problems*: Associated with your sad mood, your ability to concentrate is less (check here ☐ if true) and you feel as though your memory is poorer (check here ☐ if true).

☐ *Hopelessness*: You have been having thoughts and feelings that life is not worth living. If you have had any thoughts of ending your life, check here ☐. You should talk to your family doctor or seek professional help if you checked this last box. Always seek professional help if you check any of the following boxes:

   ☐ I have recently had thoughts of taking my life.

   ☐ I have a plan for taking my life.

   ☐ I have made preparations for taking my life.

   ☐ I have begun to say my good-byes.

   ☐ I intend to take my life soon.

Any of these feelings are dangerous warning signs—you should seek immediate help. Tell someone about these feelings *today*!

If, after reading this section, you or a loved one thinks that you are clinically depressed, what can you expect? Although many people remain reluctant to see a mental health professional for fear of being labeled, you should realize that depression is a common and treatable condition that can develop in almost anyone. There are a number of psychological and medical treatments that are highly effective for depression. Your doctor can help you decide on the best course of treatment for you and can often recommend a good psychiatrist or psychologist. Antidepressant medications are highly effective for treating most depressions, and psychotherapy (such as cognitive behavioral or interpersonal therapy) is also an effective treatment option. Above all, don't suffer silently.

Anxiety Disorders

As with depression, we all get anxious and worried at times. Indeed, anxiety is a very common factor underlying irritable bowel, as you have seen in this workbook (for those with diarrhea, fears of public appearances and lack of confidence in social situations can be a crippling problem). Yet some people are so dominated by anxiety that it interferes with many aspects of their lives. There are several subtypes of anxiety disorders: panic, generalized anxiety, obsessive-compulsive syndrome, and posttraumatic stress.

Panic refers to the sudden, intense onrush of anxiety that can't be ignored. It's like going from zero to sixty in two seconds. People who have had panic attacks usually remember them vividly. When people have repeated panic attacks that they can't predict (they occur out of the blue) and can't control, this can lead to panic disorder. If you have had two or more episodes of panic within a short period of time (one to two months) and live in fear of further panic attacks, you should see a mental health professional. A common consequence of having unexpected panic attacks is developing a pattern of avoidance: usually, people avoid any situation in which they do not feel safe. This is called *agoraphobia* and is an indication for professional treatment. People who have panic attacks may also have phobias, meaning fears of specific things. The most disabling phobia is social phobia, in which the person lives in dread of being evaluated negatively by others (you probably recall hearing that fear of public speaking is the most common fear). Other phobias include intense fear and avoidance of animals, blood, heights, water, flying, and so on. As with depression, there are a number of medical and psychological treatments that can be very effective for treating panic disorders.

Generalized anxiety refers to the tendency of some people to worry to excess about most everything (big and small) most of the time. These people are often referred to as worrywarts. All of us worry, but most of the time the things we worry about have a realistic threat attached to them. People who have generalized anxiety disorder worry about things that are minor as well as major, spend most of their time worrying, and are generally unable to control or dismiss their worries. Subjective distress and interference with normal activities are the keys to deciding whether the person worries to excess or has a generalized anxiety disorder. Often, professional advice is needed to accurately diagnose generalized anxiety. Generalized anxiety disorder is very similar to somatic preoccupation. The main difference is that with somatic preoccupation the anxiety is focused specifically on medical illnesses.

We will mention two other anxiety disorders for the sake of completeness. They are relatively uncommon and are not often associated with irritable bowel. Obsessive-compulsive disorder involves either anxiety-provoking thoughts that can't be controlled (called obsessions or ruminations) or behaviors that make no sense and are compulsively repeated (such as excessive hand washing, checking locks, counting objects, and so on). Posttraumatic stress disorder can develop after the experience of a trauma, such as being in a bad car accident, raped, robbed, assaulted, and so on. The symptoms include reliving the trauma in one's mind, general anxiety, intrusive thoughts, and feelings of detachment from life in general. If you think you may have either of these problems, talk to your family doctor about a more detailed assessment.

Substance Abuse Disorders

Finally, we would like to mention the problem of substance abuse. In an attempt to cope with life problems, such as irritable bowel, some people turn to drugs or medication. Alcohol is commonly used by men to cope with anxiety. Alcohol has a different effect in women than in men, based on differences in size and body composition. Thus, women have less tolerance for alcohol than men. Many women don't label themselves as having an alcohol problem when drinking three to four drinks per day, but this can be equivalent to six to eight drinks for a man.

Some people who are against street drugs can develop problems with prescription medication. This is especially true for managing chronic pain. Many powerful painkillers are very addictive (such as Demerol or OxyContin).

One way to determine whether you have a substance abuse problem is to ask someone you trust (who doesn't have a problem himself or herself) if he or she is concerned about your substance use. It is sometimes very difficult to identify the problem from within. There are a wide variety of effective means of reducing substance abuse problems.

Physicians are often trained to ask a series of four questions to assess the presence of a drinking problem. This is known as the CAGE assessment. The questions are printed here. If you check two or more of these questions, it is likely that you have a drinking problem and should seek help.

The CAGE Questionnaire

Check any of the boxes that are true for you. If you check two or more boxes, it is likely that you have a drinking problem and should seek help.

C ☐ Have you ever felt a need to **C**ut down on your drinking?

A ☐ Have you ever felt **A**nnoyed when people comment on your drinking?

G ☐ Have you felt **G**uilty about your drinking?

E ☐ Have you had a drink in the morning to get rid of a hangover or to steady your nerves (an **E**ye-opener)

13

Working with Your Doctor

When irritable bowel symptoms first surface, a doctor will focus on the following question: Is something dangerous causing these symptoms? Once irritable bowel is diagnosed, the focus turns to managing those symptoms and responding to any problems.

In many ways, having irritable bowel forces you to become your own doctor. It is up to you to control your symptoms, to choose what you eat, when you eat, and how you act and react to life's daily stresses. Your physician will be the person you turn to for expert advice and to decide if symptom changes warrant more tests.

Few doctors receive much training in managing irritable bowel, and most can't advise you about specific nutrition strategies (that's why this book is so important). Even so, you should contact your doctor if your symptoms change or if you experience problems not associated with irritable bowel, such as blood in the stool (see chapters 1 and 2).

To get the most from your doctor's appointments, the following are a few things to remember:

- *If you have a specific concern, tell your doctor immediately.* Some patients don't mention what's really on their minds until they are putting on their coats and heading to the door. By waiting until the last moment, your doctor may not recognize your question as a major concern or will assume you just want a quick reassurance.

- *If you are afraid you have cancer, say so.* Speaking the word *cancer* does not mean you will get it. We mention cancer specifically because it is very common for people with irritable bowel to have this fear. Doctors know the symptoms of cancer and can quickly evaluate your symptoms and provide reassurance if they do not indicate cancer. If, however, you do not express your fear about cancer (or any other symptom), your doctor will assume that you know the symptoms are not dangerous. Internalizing concerns often causes distress, which can contribute to the worsening of your symptoms. Many patients see improvement simply by being reassured that they do not have cancer, colitis, or another dangerous bowel disease.

- *Resist being intimidated by your doctor.* Doctors are often very busy and may give you the impression that they are having to rush to see you. To help avoid being flustered, try to jot down your questions so you are sure you won't forget them. It will also help to bring your symptom list from chapter 2.

- *Remember, there are no stupid questions.* Your doctor has heard them all and can most likely address any concern, but you need to voice them. Being yourself and speaking frankly about your concerns goes a long way in building a trusting relationship with your doctor. This is crucial. If you do not believe what your doctor tells you, then you will not be reassured and you will probably end up seeing other doctors unnecessarily.

- *Seek out a doctor who listens to and answers your questions and continue seeing that doctor.* Doctors know when they don't have the right skills to manage a problem and will refer you to other specialists if necessary. Seeing many doctors for second opinions usually leads to unnecessary tests, and little is done to help you manage your symptoms.

- *Make sure you understand your doctor's instructions.* If your doctor gives you advice or asks you to do something, it is important to clarify what he or she wants you to do. You should understand why you are taking a medication, what it is supposed to do, and any side effects to watch for. Only by making sure you understand your doctor's instructions will it be possible for you to work effectively with your doctor.

A Patient-Doctor Dialogue

Much of your discussion with your doctor probably will be related to the symptoms of irritable bowel. We thought it would be helpful to review what we know about these symptoms by presenting a dialogue that covers common questions and comments from patients.

Patient: When my bowels work, the stool often starts off as solid or even hard. Then it becomes increasingly loose after I have gone to the bathroom several times over an hour or two. I have severe cramps in the lower belly and often feel tired and drained. Also, I sometimes feel hot and break out in a sweat.

Doctor: Irritable bowel will frequently cause this pattern of defecation. In fact, it can be used to diagnose irritable bowel. What you have described are three of the six typical irritable bowel symptoms. You start with solid stool that becomes increasingly loose and more frequent and is associated with the abdominal cramping pain. After your bowel motion you also notice that you have a feeling of incomplete rectal emptying. And if you look at the bowel motion, you may see a slimy substance in the stool. This substance, which we call mucus, is a normal lubricant produced in the bowel. There may be times that you just pass this slimy substance with little or no stool.

You will feel tired and drained with sweating because your body has reacted to the diarrhea by activating the sympathetic nervous system. These are the nerves that prime the heart to pump blood more quickly through the body, which often causes a flushing sensation that makes you feel warm. Then you start sweating to regulate your body temperature so it does not rise with the increased blood flow to the body tissues. These are normal sensations known as the body's fight or flight response that occurs when our bodies feel threatened. The response can also occur with diarrhea or other unpleasant symptoms.

It is not in your head. These are normal body sensations even though they can feel unpleasant and alarming.

Patient: I usually feel so bloated after eating that on most days I eat just one big meal. I skip breakfast and rarely have lunch because I know eating makes the bloating worse. I am often constipated and unable to have a bowel motion more than twice a week.

Doctor: Healthy eating habits and trying to keep a routine eating schedule will be important for your bowel. Right now, you are not eating in a way that will help to improve your constipation. Breakfast is probably the most important meal of the day because your large bowel is most active in the morning when you wake up. Eating breakfast will further stimulate your bowel and greatly increase your chances of having more regular bowel motions.

Abdominal bloating tends to be worse if you eat just one meal a day, especially if it's a large meal. Bloating also tends to be worse later in the day. To help ease your bloating, try to eat smaller meals more frequently and earlier in the day. Make breakfast your larger meal of the day and supper a light snack. (For a more comprehensive guide on how to manage gas and bloating symptoms, see chapter 7.)

Patient: I've noticed undigested food when I have gone to the bathroom, especially when I have diarrhea. I am not too surprised to see corn, but sometimes I see tomato skins, seeds, or other pieces of fruits and vegetables.

Doctor: What you are describing is normal. Fibrous foods such as vegetables and fruits are not completely digested even though their nutrients are absorbed in the intestines. Undigested food is just easier to spot if you have diarrhea. Corn can be seen even in normal solid stool because of its bright yellow color, but other undigested foods are in the stool as well. It is *not* normal to see meat fibers and fat in the stool. This indicates a problem with food digestion.

At times, you may notice that the normal mucus present in stool looks like fat globules. This can be confusing, but it is rare for the body to be having trouble absorbing fat and not lose weight. If you are losing weight, further testing can be done on the stool to determine whether you have a problem with fat absorption.

Patient: I am worried that I may have a digestion problem. My stool often floats. Doesn't that mean fat isn't being digested properly?

Doctor: Most of the time a floating stool means that gas from the intestine, not fat, has been trapped in the solid stool allowing it to float. Stools that float are normal and nothing to worry about.

Patient: Sometimes when I have diarrhea my stool turns green after several bowel motions. Is this serious?

Doctor: Stool gets its normal brown color when bacteria change unabsorbed bile in the intestine to a yellow-brown pigment. If you have diarrhea, the stool can pass through the gut too quickly for this color change to occur. The only abnormal colors for stool are: red, black, and an off-white or clay-colored stool. Light-colored stools can be due to bile not getting into the intestines in the first place. This is usually accompanied by jaundice (a yellow color to the skin and the whites of the eyes) and urine that is dark yellow or almost brown (tea colored). Stool that is red or black can be due to internal bleeding and blood loss. The source of a red color is obvious; the black color occurs because bacteria in the gut change the red color in blood to a black pigment. Tests can be done on the stool if it is black to determine if there is blood present.

Further tests should always be done if the stool is red or black to find the cause of bleeding. Bleeding is not normal and is not part of irritable bowel. Some causes of bleeding can be minor, such as hemorrhoids or an anal fissure (a split or tear in the skin lining the anal opening to the rectum). You should always tell your doctor if you see bleeding so that the true cause can be found.

Some medications can also turn the bowel motions black. The most common is iron medication, but if you are taking iron for anemia or "low blood," tests should first be done to check the stool for blood (even if the stool has a normal brown color) to be sure the anemia is not due to blood loss from the gut. Licorice and medications with bismuth such as Pepto-Bismol can also cause a black discoloration of the stool.

Patient: I have been looking up information on IBS on the Internet. I found one medication that is made of "all natural ingredients" and that will regulate my bowels. I have also been reading information that claims that IBS is a mental disorder, not a real disease.

Doctor: When seeking out further information, particularly on the Internet, you should be very careful about the claims of products for treating medical conditions. Many "all-natural ingredients" claims for products that "help" the bowels work often contain laxatives that are classed as stimulants. These come from plant extracts, and the most common ones are Senna and Cascara sagrada, which can actually damage the bowel and aggravate constipation if taken daily for long periods of time. The manufacturer can correctly claim the product is "all natural" since it is the extract from the plants that have laxative properties in the bowel. But other plants, such as nightshade, could also carry the healthy sounding "all natural" label, yet are known to be deadly poisons. If you plan to buy such products, it is as always, buyer beware! If you are not sure, bring in the ingredient list and we can check it over to see if there are any potentially harmful substances in the product.

As for the information you may find on the Internet, remember that anyone can put information on the Internet, even if it is incorrect. People used to think that irritable bowel was a psychological disorder. We now know that this is incorrect. Psychological factors such as stress and anxiety will worsen your irritable bowel, but they are not the cause of your symptoms.

14

Living with Irritable Bowel

We truly hope that you have found this book useful. But before you return it to its place on the shelf, we have two suggestions.

First, sit down and write yourself a letter. That's right, write a letter to yourself! Let us explain. We want you to write a letter to the person you were before starting this book. Knowing what you do now, advise yourself on how to handle irritable bowel. Identify the symptoms you began with and how they were distressing to you. Go on to list what you have learned about those symptoms and your body. Identify your dietary and psychological triggers, and then tell yourself what interventions you found helpful (and how you implemented them). Then put this letter inside the front cover of this book.

If sometime in the future (six months or six years) you begin to experience irritable bowel again, reread the letter. We have found that if you capture in your own words your experience in treating irritable bowel, it will be tremendously helpful should you need to treat yourself again in the future. Combined with using this book, you should be in good shape to prevent future problems.

The second thing we suggest is that you complete another symptoms diary, as you did in chapter 2. We supply an extra diary form on the following pages. Once you have completed the diary again, compare it to your first one. Not only will this show you how far you have come but it will also point out remaining issues that may need special attention in the future.

One final point: We thought you might find it useful if we listed what we feel are the top ten things to do to manage irritable bowel. We hope you find the list helpful.

The Top Ten Tips for Living with Irritable Bowel

1. Remember that your bowel is normal—just "irritable."
2. Your bowel will thrive on routine (eat meals regularly and get adequate sleep).
3. Identify and limit foods that trigger symptoms.
4. Eat plenty of fiber (20 to 35 grams daily for people with constipation or an alternating bowel habit) and drink 8 eight-ounce glasses of caffeine-free liquid each day.
5. Adjust your food choices and habits to your symptoms.
6. Identify sources of stress.
7. Practice stress management strategies.
8. Set your priorities realistically.
9. Accept, adapt, and let go.
10. Work with your doctor and express your concerns.

Thank you for taking the time to work through this book. It is our hope that we have empowered you to reduce the control that irritable bowel symptoms can have on your life.

SYMPTOMS DIARY

	Symptoms (note time as well)	Severity of Symptoms (1 = minimal/negligible; 10 = extreme severity)	Food Triggers (that is, foods eaten *before* symptoms)	Stress Level (1 = no stress; 10 = extreme stress)	Feelings and Worries
Monday					
Tuesday					
Wednesday					

(continued)

187

SYMPTOMS DIARY *(continued)*

	Symptoms (note time as well)	Severity of Symptoms (1 = minimal/negligible; 10 = extreme severity)	Food Triggers (that is, foods eaten *before* symptoms)	Stress Level (1 = no stress; 10 = extreme stress)	Feelings and Worries
Thursday					
Friday					
Saturday					
Sunday					

APPENDIX

High-Fiber, Low-Fat Recipes

Before presenting a few high-fiber, low-fat recipes, the following are some pointers on how to increase the fiber and reduce the fat content in existing recipes.

To increase the fiber (insoluble) content:

- Use half whole wheat and half white flour in baked items.
- Add natural bran to pancakes, muffins, cakes, hot cereal, stews, casseroles, soups, and meatloaf.
- Choose whole wheat pasta instead of pasta made with white flour.

To decrease the fat content:

- Decrease the fat in your recipes by a third to a half. For example, a muffin recipe that calls for ½ cup of margarine can be cut back to ¼ cup with little, if any, change in the finished product.
- Add moisture to recipes by adding fruit like applesauce or canned pumpkin. Applesauce does not add flavor. By adding applesauce and pumpkin, you can cut back on the sugar in the recipe as well. Adding fruit may extend the cooking time by two to three minutes.
- Reduce fat, saturated fat, and cholesterol in your recipes by decreasing the egg yolk content by half. For example, if a recipe calls for two whole eggs, use one whole egg and one egg white.

The following recipes were developed mostly from existing recipes using the foregoing guidelines. While the recipes are reduced in fat and have added fiber, some do not meet the strict definition of low fat (3 grams of fat per serving) or high fiber (5 grams or more of fiber per serving).

Metric Conversion Chart

½ tsp = 2 ml

1 tsp = 5 ml

2 tsp = 10 ml

1 Tbsp = 15 ml

¼ cup = 60 ml

⅓ cup = 75 ml

½ cup = 120 ml

⅔ cup = 150 ml

¾ cup = 175 ml

1 cup = 250 ml

1¼ cups = 300 ml

1½ cups = 375 ml

Grainy Gingerbread Cake

½	cup packed brown sugar
¼	cup margarine
1	egg
1	egg white
1	cup unsweetened applesauce
½	cup molasses
¾	cup whole wheat flour
¾	cup all-purpose flour
½	cup natural (baker's) bran
1	teaspoon baking soda
1	teaspoon baking powder
2	teaspoons ground ginger
1	teaspoon cinnamon
1	teaspoon salt

fruit-flavored low-fat yogurt (optional)

In a bowl, using an electric mixer, beat the brown sugar and margarine until smooth. Add the egg and egg white, beating well after each addition. Add the applesauce and molasses; beat until smooth. In a separate bowl, combine the flour, natural bran, baking soda, baking powder, ginger, cinnamon, and salt; gradually beat into the sugar and egg mixture, beating for 2–3 minutes. Transfer to an 8-inch lightly greased and floured square cake pan. Bake at 350 degrees F for 40 minutes. Pour the fruit-flavored low-fat yogurt over the gingerbread before serving.

Makes 12 servings

Per serving (cake only): Calories 170, carbohydrates 31 g, protein 2 g, fat 4 g, saturated fat 1 g, cholesterol 18 mg, fiber 2.3 g

Irish Soda Bread

2	cups whole wheat flour
1	cup white flour
1	cup natural bran
1	cup quick cooking oats
1½	teaspoons baking soda
1	teaspoon baking powder
1	teaspoon salt
2	tablespoons sesame seeds (optional)
3	tablespoons poppy seeds (optional)
¼	cup liquid honey
2	cups buttermilk or low-fat plain yogurt

In a bowl, mix the flour, bran, oats, baking soda, baking powder, salt, and seeds. Combine the honey with the dry ingredients. Make a well in the center of the mixture. Add the buttermilk or yogurt and mix until fully combined. Pour into a pie plate. Make a cross on the top of the dough with the sharp edge of a knife. Bake at 375 degrees F for 40–50 minutes.

Makes 16 servings

Per serving: Calories 155, carbohydrates 35 g, protein 5.8 g, fat 3 g, saturated fat 0.5 g, cholesterol 1 mg, fiber 4.2 g

Whole Wheat Pizza Crust

2	teaspoons sugar
2	cups warm water
2	envelopes fast-rise yeast
1/4	cup vegetable oil
2 1/2	cups whole wheat flour
2	cups white flour

Dissolve the sugar in the warm water in a large bowl. Sprinkle the yeast into the water and let it stand 10 minutes. Stir the oil into the yeast mixture. Stir in half of the whole wheat flour. Then add the remaining whole wheat and white flours, mixing until the dough can be gathered in a slightly sticky ball. On a lightly floured surface, knead the dough for about 5 minutes or until smooth and elastic. Cut the dough in half, cover with waxed paper, and let it rest for 30–40 minutes. On a floured surface, roll out each piece of dough to about 12 inches in diameter. Transfer to a lightly greased pizza round and carefully pull and stretch with your fingers to make it fit the pan. Let the dough rest for about 20–30 minutes more before adding toppings. For a thicker crust, let the dough rest for 30–40 minutes. Spread with tomato sauce, your favorite vegetables, and low-fat cheese just before baking. Bake at 450 degrees F for 15–20 minutes.

Makes two 12-inch pizza rounds.

Total of 16 servings; each serving equals 1/8 of one pizza

Per serving: Calories 159, carbohydrates 36 g, protein 4.2 g, fat 4 g, saturated fat 0.6 g, cholesterol 0 g, fiber 2.8 g

Nan's Cookies

$^2/_3$	cup soft margarine
1	cup white sugar
2	large eggs
$^1/_4$	cup milk
$1^1/_2$	cups quick cooking oats
1	cup white flour
$^1/_2$	cup natural wheat bran
1	cup whole wheat flour
1	teaspoon cinnamon
1	teaspoon baking soda
1	teaspoon baking powder
1	teaspoon salt
$^1/_2$	cup raisins
$^1/_2$	cup chopped dates

Beat the margarine and sugar together until smooth. Beat in the eggs, one at a time. Add the milk. In a separate bowl, combine the oats, flours, bran, cinnamon, baking soda, baking powder, salt, raisins, and dates. Add the dry ingredients to the liquid mixture and mix well. Drop by large tablespoons onto a baking sheet. Bake at 350 degrees F for 15 minutes.

Makes 3 dozen cookies

Per serving: Calories 120, carbohydrates 19 g, protein 2.2 g, fat 4.5 g, saturated fat 0.85 g, cholesterol 12 mg, fiber 1.7 g

Oat and Wheat Bran Muffins with Fruit

1	egg
³⁄₄	cup 1% milk
¹⁄₃	cup vegetable oil
¹⁄₂	cup unsweetened applesauce (optional)
1	apple, chopped
¹⁄₂	cup dried cranberries
¹⁄₂	cup raisins
¹⁄₂	cup quick cooking oats
¹⁄₂	cup natural wheat bran
¹⁄₂	cup white flour
¹⁄₂	cup whole wheat flour
¹⁄₃	cup sugar
1	tablespoon baking powder
1	teaspoon salt
1	teaspoon nutmeg
2	teaspoons cinnamon

Beat the egg, and combine with the milk, oil, and applesauce. In a separate bowl, combine the apple, cranberries, raisins, oats, bran, flours, sugar, baking power, salt, nutmeg, and cinnamon. Add the liquid ingredients to the dry ingredients and stir until well mixed. Fill 12 muffin cups with the mixture. Bake at 400 degrees F for 20 minutes.

Makes 12 muffins

Per serving: Calories 200, carbohydrates 28 g, protein 2.8 g, fat 8 g,
    saturated fat 0.18 g, cholesterol 212 mg, fiber 3.4 g

Pumpkin Bran Muffins

- ¼ cup vegetable oil
- ½ cup brown sugar
- ¼ cup molasses
- 1 egg
- 1 egg white
- ¾ cup 1% milk
- 1 cup canned pumpkin
- 1¼ cups white flour
- 1½ teaspoons baking powder
- ½ teaspoon baking soda
- ¾ teaspoon salt
- 1½ cups natural wheat bran
- ½ cup raisins

Mix together the vegetable oil, brown sugar, and molasses. Add the egg and egg white, beating after each addition. Stir in the milk and canned pumpkin. In a separate bowl, combine the flour, baking powder, baking soda, salt, bran, and raisins. Combine the liquid and dry ingredients, mixing as little as possible. Fill lightly greased muffin cups ¾ full. Bake at 400 degrees F for 17–20 minutes.

Makes 12 muffins

Per serving: Calories 193, carbohydrates 45.6 g, protein 3.4 g, fat 5.7 g, saturated fat 0.1 g, cholesterol 18 mg, fiber 4.4 g

High-Fiber Chocolate Muffins

1   440 gram package low-fat fudge brownie mix

1½ teaspoons baking soda

3   cups very-high-fiber cereal (more than10 grams per ½ cup)

2½ cups boiling water

Pour the boiling water over the cereal and mix until combined. Let it cool for approximately 15 minutes. Mix the baking soda with the brownie mix. Combine the cereal-water mixture with the brownie mix until well combined. Fill 12 muffin cups ¾ full. Bake at 350 degrees F for 20–25 minutes.

Makes 12 muffins

Per serving: Calories 207, carbohydrates 10.6 g, protein 4.5 g, fat 6 g,
    saturated fat 0.15 g, cholesterol 0 g, fiber 6 g

Blueberry Whole-Wheat Pancakes

1   cup white flour

1   cup whole wheat flour

¼   teaspoon cinnamon

½   teaspoon salt

1½   cups 1% milk

2   tablespoons vegetable oil

1   egg

1   cup blueberries

Mix together the flours, cinnamon, and salt. In a separate bowl, beat together the milk, oil, and egg, and add to the dry ingredients. Blend until there are no lumps. Refrigerate for a couple of hours or overnight. When you are ready to make the pancakes, stir in the blueberries. Brush a skillet or griddle with oil or use a nonstick pan. Set the burner to medium. Pour the batter using ¼ cup for each pancake. When the underside is brown and bubbles break on the top (after 1 or 2 minutes), turn the pancake over and cook for 30–60 seconds or until the other side is golden brown.

Makes 12 servings

Per serving: Calories 118, carbohydrates 27 g, protein 3.5 g, fat 3.4 g, saturated fat 0.7 g, cholesterol 185 mg, fiber 1.8 g

Vegetarian Lasagna

1	tablespoon vegetable oil
1	small onion, chopped
3	cloves garlic, finely chopped
2	carrots, chopped
2	cups sliced mushrooms
1	19-ounce can tomatoes
1	7½-ounce can tomato sauce
2	teaspoons dried basil
2	teaspoons dried oregano
salt and freshly ground pepper	
1	12 oz. package frozen spinach, thawed, chopped
9	whole wheat lasagna noodles
1	cup low-fat cottage cheese
3	cups shredded low-fat mozzarella cheese
⅓	cup grated Parmesan cheese
¾	teaspoon hot sauce (optional)

Heat the oil on medium heat in a large saucepan. Add the onion and cook until soft. Stir in the garlic, carrots, and mushrooms. Cook, stirring often, for 5 minutes. Add the tomatoes. Break up the mixture with a fork. Stir in the tomato sauce, basil, and oregano; season with the salt and pepper to taste. Simmer uncovered for 10 minutes or until slightly thickened. Add the chopped spinach. Let the mixture cool. In large pot of boiling water, cook the noodles until tender but firm; drain and rinse under cold water. In a lightly greased 13-by-9-inch baking dish, arrange three noodles evenly over the bottom. Spread ½ of the vegetable mixture, then ½ of the cottage cheese. Sprinkle with ⅓ of the mozzarella cheese. Repeat the noodle, vegetable mixture, cottage cheese, and mozzarella cheese layers once. Arrange the remaining noodles over the top; sprinkle with the remaining mozzarella cheese and the Parmesan cheese. Bake at 350 degrees for 35–45 minutes or until hot and bubbly.

Makes 8 servings

Per serving: Calories 332, carbohydrates 37 g, protein 22 g, fat 11 g, saturated fat 5.5 g, cholesterol 30 mg, fiber 5 g

Pasta with Tomato and Feta

1	pound whole wheat penne noodles
1	tablespoon olive oil
2	cloves garlic, finely chopped
4	large plum tomatoes, cut into wedges
$\frac{1}{3}$	cup black olives, halved
$\frac{1}{2}$	cup crumbled feta cheese
$\frac{1}{2}$	cup chopped fresh parsley
2	teaspoons dried basil
$\frac{1}{4}$	cup grated Parmesan cheese

In a large pot of boiling water, cook the noodles until tender but firm. Drain and keep warm. Heat the oil in a large nonstick skillet. Stir in the garlic. Add the tomatoes and cook, stirring for 3 minutes or until heated through. Combine with the drained pasta. Add the olives, feta cheese, parsley, and basil; toss gently to mix. Sprinkle with the Parmesan cheese.

Makes 4 main-course servings

Per serving: Calories 609, carbohydrates 96 g, protein 23 g, fat 15 g, saturated fat 9 g, cholesterol 32 mg, fiber 7 g

INDEX

abdominal pain
  healthy eating adjustments for,
    84–85
  pain medication and, 155–56,
    178, 183, 184
  See also pain
abuse
  physical, 13, 157
  substance, 177–78
acid, 28
  antireflux diet for, 87–88, 100,
    107–10
  benefits of, 29
  See also heartburn
Africans, lactose intolerance in,
  112
age, of irritable bowel onset, 8–9
agoraphobia, 176
air swallowing, 30, 86–87
alcohol, 110–11
  abuse of, 177–78
  CAGE Questionnaire, 178
  heartburn and, 109–10
antidepressants, 155–56
antireflux diet
  description of, 107–10
  indications for, 87
  vitamin supplements for, 100
antispasm drugs, 156
anxiety, 23, 169

disorders, 176–77
  reassurance and, 173
  somatic preoccupation and, 171
  See also psychological factors
apple body shape, 62–63
applesauce
  in Grainy Gingerbread Cake, 191
  in Oat and Wheat Bran Muffins
    with Fruit, 195
  to reduce fat in recipes, 189
Asians
  lactose intolerance in, 112
  waist circumference guidelines
    for, 63
assertiveness, 141, 142
  broken record technique, 142–43
  fogging technique, 143–47

bacteria, probiotics, 41
beans, 49, 53, 55
behavior. *See* lifestyle; psychological factors
beta carotene, 99
bile salts, 32–33
black-and-white thinking, 139
bloating
  air swallowing and, 30, 86–87
  healthy eating adjustments for,
    84
  low gassy foods diet for, 95–101

CPSIA information can be obtained at www.ICGtesting.com
Printed in the USA
BVOW02n2049010514

352303BV00007B/14/P